Praise for The Actual Dance

"This beautiful book is a poignant reminder of all we take for granted in our lives. This book will cause you to think differently and more deeply about the day-to-day interactions with the one you love most in your life and certainly cause you to hug that person just a little tighter."

—**William Kennard,**
chairman of AT&T's board of directors, former U.S. Ambassador to the European Union, former chair of the Federal Communications Commission

"The Actual Dance is beautiful, powerful, and timeless in its messages. I hope this is very widely read and absorbed."

—**James Fallows,**
award-winning and bestseller author, contributing writer at *The Atlantic,* a former editor of *U.S. News & World Report*

"Written from the perspective of a husband whose wife was just diagnosed with cancer. Sam describes his journey with the metaphor of a dance, 'The Actual Dance,' that is controlling his mind. A must-read."

—**Eileen Robin Filler-Corn,**
56th Speaker of the Virginia House of Delegates, lawyer, former advisor to U.S. Senator Mark Warner

"A rarely heard voice in the breast cancer journey. Sam gives voice to the depth of his love and fear of loss. The story itself is a metaphor for a ritual we know will come. It is a story of what love really means."

—**Congressman Gerry Connelly,**
U.S. Representative from Virginia's 11th congressional district, former chair of the Fairfax County Board of Supervisors.

"In *The Actual Dance*, Sam Simon weaves together the fascinating story behind his writing and producing a play of the same name with the real-life events he experienced while confronting his wife Susan's cancer. The integration of these two realities strengthens the poignancy of each, and we, the readers, benefit profoundly. With intimate detail, Sam recounts the oft-untold emotional roller coaster of the caregivers who endure the life-threatening illness of a loved one. The story is universal, and I highly recommend it for everyone."

—**Reverend Robert Chase,**
former director of communications for United Church of Christ, founding director of Intersections International, award-winning video producer and director

"When a born pessimist falls for a born optimist, they experience life's trials and triumphs together. When said optimist Susan gets serious breast cancer, Sam must face his biggest fears. Will he dance alone in his dream waltz of despair, or will Susan's grit and grace beat his demons? This startling memoir is a celebration of love and hope, where the sick heal the caretaker and the caretaker learns humility and happiness."

—**Rabbi Naamah Kelman,**
Dean of the Hebrew Union College-Jewish Institute
of Religion campus in Jerusalem, Israel

"*The Actual Dance* is a dialogue of great sensitivity and emotional complexity of a man and his struggles dealing with the most important women in his life who were diagnosed with breast cancer—his wife, his mother and his mother-in-law—and with their survival and/or death. In this book, the true impact of the diagnosis of his wife's breast cancer is often hidden in the deep recesses of his emotions and his life. The dance is a metaphor for the swirling in and of his life. Anyone who reads this book will be profoundly affected."

—**Richard Binder,**
M. D., acclaimed metal sculptor
and retired oncologist

"Through the terror of a dreaded cancer diagnosis, *The Actual Dance* is a poignant love story bearing witness to all its messiness. Sam's experience of his wife Susan's breast cancer explores the power of hope to overcome despair. It's a tender story of navigating the dimensions of fear, punctuated by optimism, to overcome the unimaginable odds."

—Roberta Baskin,
award-winning investigative journalist,
co-founder and former executive director of the
AIM2Flourish global learning initiative

"Sam Simon has written a brilliant book addressing a subject that few have visited—the role of caregiver (or, as Sam self-identifies, 'love partner') to his devoted wife of more than 30 years, who has just received a bad breast cancer diagnosis. As the prognosis becomes more dire, Sam finds himself transported to a hall with a full orchestra playing the couple's favorite song, 'the actual dance' of the title. This is a book for anyone who has ever loved and desires to grasp a fuller understanding of what that love truly means."

—Frances Schwartz,
educator in Jewish Studies,
co-author of *Jewish Moral Virtues* and
A Touch of the Sacred, author of *Passage to Pesach*.

"The world of family caregiving has many, many different faces. It is not just caring for grandma and grandpa. Sam Simon invites us into a world few have been brave enough to articulate: His journey, yes, his journey, through his wife's breast cancer. It is a powerful and power-filled production, and now this wonderful book is full of even more details. I feel so blessed to have been invited to *The Actual Dance*... Join us, go deeply into the dance of a lifetime."

—Reverend Gregory Johnson,
president & CEO, Greg Johnson Partnerships International, Inc., former director at Emblem Health, New York, the Care for the Family Caregiver program

the Actual Dance

SAMUEL A. SIMON

For Marc,
a true mensch! May
all your work be a blessing to
the world. Thank you!
Samuel A Simon
11-24-2021

The Actual Dance: Love's Ultimate Journey Through Cancer

Disclaimer

This is a work of creative non-fiction. All information provided in this book is for general informational and entertainment purposes. The events and conversations in this memoir are true to the best of the author's memory *and not a source of medical or other advice*. The author and publisher assume no responsibility for errors, inaccuracies, omissions, or any other inconsistencies herein. The medical information and treatments are as recalled by the author, a writer, and should not be viewed as medically accurate either at the time referred to in the book, or as advice or basis for a modern treatment of breast cancer. *Anyone who suspects they have cancer or any other illness should seek immediate medical attention by qualified medical personnel.*

For information about this title or to order other books and/or electronic media, contact the publisher:

The Actual Dance, LLC
McLean, Virginia
info@theactualdance.com

Paperback ISBN: 978-1-7379097-0-5
Hardcover ISBN: 978-1-7379097-2-9
eBook ISBN: 978-1-7379097-1-2

Publisher's Cataloging-In-Publication Data
(Prepared by The Donohue Group, Inc.)
Names: Simon, Sam, 1945- author. | Simon, Sam, 1945- Actual dance (Play)
Title: The actual dance : love's ultimate journey through breast cancer / Samuel A. Simon.
Description: [Mclean, Virginia] : The Actual Dance, LLC, [2021] | Based on the author's play, The actual dance.
Identifiers: ISBN 9781737909705 (paperback) | ISBN 9781737909729 (hardcover) | ISBN 9781737909712 (ebook)
Subjects: LCSH: Simon, Sam, 1945---Marriage. | Breast--Cancer--Psychological aspects. | Breast--Cancer--Patients--Family relationships. | Married people. | Love.
Classification: LCC RC280.B8 S56 2021 (print) | LCC RC280.B8 (ebook) | DDC 362.19699449--dc23

Printed in the United States of America

To

Susan Meryl Kalmans Simon
The other half of my whole

Preface

As you move through this book, I hope you suspend disbelief, let go of all your assumptions, and discover for yourself places of boundless love in your life. If I could, I would whisper in your ear from time to time as you make your way through these pages. I would gently assure you, "Yes, it is true. It exists! The places, the moments, and the love are all real."

The story and every moment in this book happened. You will learn all the details of two young people who meet, fall in love, and grow up together as a married couple. This part of the story will be familiar, maybe mundane, though I hope engaging. "It," though, is something else. "It" is a different place in time and space to which I travel seamlessly and simultaneously as I stand on the edge of the abyss. The experience suggests an answer to how I came to terms with the anticipated loss of the love of my life, Susan.

As my whispers would assure you, this book is not fiction. While I changed a few names to protect the privacy of a few individuals, the incidents, the moments of boundary-crossing, the paranormal moments are not products of the imagination. I experienced them. I assert and believe to my core that they were not hallucinations.

This memoir stems from *The Actual Dance,* a play written in 2012 and first performed in 2013. Since then, I have presented *The Actual* Dance hundreds of times at dozens of venues. With each performance, I gain new insights into my own experience of Susan's illness, which now has become this book.

This story will have a familiar ring. Many books by men focus on their caregiver role for someone, perhaps a wife, husband, or friend, with cancer. There are also many books about the end-of-life journey with a loved one. I believe this book is a little different. It defines a new and different role—beyond and distinct from that of caregiver—the role of LovePartner^{SM}.

A LovePartner^{SM} is a person whose heart and soul are breaking as they experience, or anticipate, the loss of their beloved. In this role, we are not nurses, though nurses are also indispensable players who take care—give care. There are family caregivers, and there are professional caregivers for people who are sick. Maybe the best way to explain this, and perhaps you will see it as you read—I am both a caregiver and a LovePartner^{SM}. How do you hold the one you love most in the world as they take their last breath? And how do you help your wife as she becomes sick to her stomach, or when her care requires that you give her a daily injection?

Through this journey, I came to understand that "love," as I use the word, is about a spiritual connection with another human being. It consists of knitting together over time the essence of two individuals into a singular spiritual unit. One might argue, and I do, that this "essence" is a part of a shared soul. Death rends us apart.

To be clear, Susan did not die. I do not know what the experience will be like if she predeceases me. I still consider that possibility as my worst fear. What I do know is what it feels like for that to almost happen. To await what seemed like an inevitability. To screw up my courage to do the unthinkable and hold Susan as she takes her last breath. In anticipation of that precise moment, I crossed a boundary—the boundary of the known into an ecstatic place that contained all the pieces needed for me to hold her and grant her the peace and knowledge of infinite love as she transitioned to the unknown.

My goal in telling this story is that you too might discover, when the time comes, the gift and privilege of being a LovePartner[SM].

US

Life exists within each of us as a form of the Divine.

A tangible essence of who we are.

Love is when our essence became entwined.

Each an equal half of the other.

"I love you," simply awakens the **US** in you and me.

The Actual Dance

*T*here is a dance, a dance that one day each and every one of us will dance. The dance takes place in a grand ballroom with a fabulous orchestra. The orchestra, I think, plays whatever song the dancers themselves want to hear. Even though I have been to dozens of these events and have the routine down pat, I can't recall a single tune ever played by one of these orchestras.

It might even be true that only the dancers themselves recognize the song the orchestra is playing.

You see, you can attend one of these events as a guest of the dancers. Or you might just end up in the gallery, watching as someone you know is dancing. You do not get to dance yourself, though, until it is your turn, or you are invited to be the dance partner of someone you love.

When it is my turn, I want to dance with the person I love most in the world. If it is her turn first, I want to be her dance partner, and I want us to dance a waltz. A slow, elegant, flowing, beautiful waltz. We stand in perfect form, bodies touching, and at the first note of our favorite song, we begin the ultimate journey through space and time as she dissolves into eternity.

Now, this dance is no small production, mind you. And the ballroom is no ordinary ballroom. It has vaulted ceilings with a beautiful, long, highly polished, blond-wood dance floor. Brilliant spotlights overhead create a precise bubble of light over that dance floor. A platform off to the side is large enough to hold a good-sized orchestra of forty or fifty or even more musicians.

The spotlights are so precisely focused on just the dance floor that the floor itself seems to disappear into the blackness of the ballroom. Standing in the center of the dance floor, looking off into the darkness of the ballroom, the dancers can just make out the silhouettes of people. Of all of the people they have ever met, have ever known, and have ever loved in their entire lives, ready to watch the couple dance the actual dance.

Even though there are billions of people on this earth, and even though there must be hundreds of thousands of these rituals every day, each dance is unique—designed, if you will, for the individual dancers.

However, the orchestra does not even exist until it is needed, and as it is needed, somehow the musicians know. The orchestra begins to form as each musician, an instrument in hand, appears, waiting to be called into a specific ballroom.

The musicians then enter the ballroom to which they are called, winding their way through those shadowy figures of a lifetime surrounding the dance floor. One-by-one they appear, *suddenly popping out of the darkness into the dazzling lights, walking slowly across the dance floor, mounting the orchestral platform. A violin, a cello, a bass, a clarinet, a flute followed by a piccolo, then another clarinet, and even a large harp— on and on until all the musicians are seated. They open their cases and take out their instruments in what seems like slow motion.*

Then the room fills with the familiar cacophony of an orchestra warming up before a performance.

At any point in this ritual, it is not too late. The end is not yet determined. The orchestra, even in the middle of a warm-up, can suddenly stop. The musicians return their instruments to their cases and exit the ballroom—a false alarm.

If it is not a false alarm, then the orchestra finishes its warmup and begins to play that song the dancers themselves wanted to hear and which only they recognize. The Actual Dance begins. It can be wonderful, and intimate, and beautiful. As the breathing slows and becomes shallow, the sound builds, and the dance intensifies. The breathing slows and softens even more, and the dance becomes more intense, and even more intense, and then even more intense! And then it stops. The dance ends. The music ends. It is as if the world itself has ended. The musicians pack up their instruments and dissolve into the darkness of the ballroom, disappearing until they are needed somewhere else. The ballroom sits achingly, intolerably empty, silent—almost in black and white—hollow.

CHAPTER 1

In The Beginning

I find myself in the Ballroom, standing alone in the center of its dance floor more often now. At first, I wonder if this place is real or just a figment of my imagination. In any case, this ethereal place is where the story begins, and perhaps it is fair to say, where the story ends.

My sense of this other place starts as an inkling, perhaps a premonition, in the early winter of 2000. As winter fades into spring, our life together—Susan and Sam's—is routine in the last half of our thirty-fourth year of marriage.

Indeed, life is good. If we were to stop and think about it, we would notice that we are in a perfect time of our lives. All the ups and downs of a married couple seem to be behind us. There were moments when the grass looked greener, and life choices seemed insufficient. Yet, we worked through them. Today, these challenges are in the past. Our kids, thank goodness, are no longer teenagers. Marcus is a lawyer now, married to a beautiful young woman who happens to share the name of his sister, Rachel (spelled differently) née Goldstein, now Simon. Our daughter, Rachael, is in residency to become a pediatric dentist. Susan and I are also at the top of our respective career paths and succeeding as we should. Yes, a perfect time of our life.

"Perfect" ends on a Tuesday evening shortly after I arrive home from work. I pull my leased Lincoln Town Car into the two-car garage of our beautiful home in Mclean, Virginia. I open the inside door and stride directly into the kitchen.

Susan greets me. "Hey, Sam, Great news! The doctor says everything is just fine."

My wife often starts talking as if in mid-conversation. It takes me a beat or two to catch up with her. *Ah, yes, she had her annual physical this morning.* It had not been on my mind, and I had not even gotten a "Hi, honey, how was your day?" Maddie and Lucky, our two dogs, seem more excited to see me than Susan, who slowly works her way around the dogs to give me a routine welcome-home peck on the cheek. I turn toward the fridge to grab an apple, my pre-dinner snack. Susan turns away to set the table for dinner.

She stops short, does a quick about-face, and says, "Oh, just one more thing, Sam."

A classic Columbo moment pops into my head. In the TV series featuring a disheveled detective named Columbo, the actor in a signature move always stops on his way out the door to turn back, looks at the suspect, and says, "Just one more thing, ma'am."

Susan does her version. "Oh, and just one more thing, Sam. Doctor Collins wants me to have a surgeon check out something she felt in my right breast." She points with her left hand to an area below her armpit where the chest and breast meet. "She doesn't think there's a problem. It just felt funny to her."

Susan then swings back around and continues her stride out of the kitchen, leaving me about to chomp on my pre-dinner apple as if nothing just happened.

"Susan! Stop! What are you talking about!" I step after her, put my hands on her shoulder, and turn her to face me. She looks up at me. I'm 6' 2", she is 5' 2". In that instant, I experience a soul-level shudder that is new and catches my attention. Just an "uh, oh" feeling that is fleeting and yet real enough for Susan to recognize a slight change in me. She rolls her eyes.

"Relax, Sam. Everything is fine. It just felt funny to her. The breast surgeon can decide if it needs a closer look."

Breast cancer has been a constant presence in our lives since the death of Susan's mother, and then my mother, from metastasized breast cancer. We have monitored Susan's breasts ever since we were married thirty-four years ago. If this surgeon decides to perform a biopsy, it will be Susan's fourth. Although the last one delivered some scary moments, the final judgment on each one has been the same—no cancer.

"Got it," I say, my hands still on Susan's shoulders. "Don't worry. Remember you had a mammogram just two months ago, and it was normal." Susan has been getting annual mammograms for most of her adult life.

Staring down at her brown eyes, thinking about breasts, and wanting to reassure her—or maybe me—I say, "Here, let me see if I feel anything." I reach over for not just a small feel of her right breast. She sees the sparkle in my eye, the wink. Dinner can wait. Humor and sex fix everything.

Susan's internist refers her to a new breast surgeon, Dr. John J. Morgan. It has been years since her last biopsy. We can tell that everything will be different the minute we walk into his modern, large, and very busy offices. The receptionist has all the paperwork ready when we announce ourselves. A nurse comes out to walk Susan back to a standard exam room while I sit out front. When the breast exam is over, I join Susan and Dr. Morgan in his office.

The first thing I notice is how young he looks. Yet, all the local magazines already have him rated as one of the top breast surgeons in the Washington DC area. He exudes confidence. He walks with a swagger, smiles all the time, and never seems worried. I eventually nickname him "Dr. Happy" because he is always so frigging optimistic.

"I did feel *something* during my examination," he says. "I understand what the internist meant about the area of the breast feeling different."

Then he starts asking questions. "Tell me about your family, Susan," he probes. "Any history of cancer?"

Susan tells him about her mother's breast cancer.

"Better safe than sorry. Let's take a closer look. I'll have the office schedule a biopsy."

A not unexpected result. Dr. Morgan will perform this biopsy as an out-patient procedure in one of these modern surgical centers now found in shopping malls everywhere. Much different from Susan's last three needle biopsies, all done in the doctors' offices.

Susan is not concerned. Lots of time has passed since that last biopsy, and we have a good record: zero for three. She is always optimistic: "Why should I worry, Sam, if I can't do anything about it. If the tissue tests positive for breast cancer, we'll deal with it then."

The C-word, spoken aloud, does little to calm my growing sense of alarm.

"It's going to be fine, Sam," she insists.

A week later, Susan and I step off the elevator directly into a bustling waiting room. Eight in the morning, no less. We walk up to the registration desk, sign in, fill out the paperwork, take a seat in the crowded room, and wait for Susan's turn for what seems like forever.

Twenty minutes pass before the far door opens, and a nurse pokes her head out and calls Susan's name. I can tell Susan is anxious. As she hears her name, she pops up and walks boldly toward the nurse and the half-open door. We don't even kiss. I stare at the door as she and the nurse disappear into the room. The thought pops into my mind for a nanosecond that maybe Susan won't come out. I shake it off and get back to the book I brought to read.

The wait agitates me. I stop reading, fidget, look through magazines, watch the TV tuned to some channel that plays old soap operas. Maybe something has happened. Or they've uncovered a medical problem. I often catastrophize things, immediately dreaming up the worst possible explanation.

Finally, finally: "Mr. Simon!" I jump up and head toward the nurse. "Right this way."

She leads me into a seemingly endless medical room. I look to the left and see an area filled with idle machines almost blocking a staging area for nurses and doctors working on who-knows-what. We move away from them, to the right, and walk to the back of a chair where Susan sits fully reclined with an IV drip still pinned into her right arm. Eyes open. Parched lips. She is loopy from the mild sedative they've given her.

I sit in the chair on the opposite side. Susan stares at the glass of water on the table across from me, her mouth slightly open, and licks her lips. She wants a drink. I stand and reach over to hold it for her to sip.

I start to fidget again as we wait for the doctor to arrive with the results. At first, I suppress my instinct to assume the worst. The staff might just need to let him know we are ready, or maybe he has another patient or two. That might explain the delay.

The clock keeps ticking. *Where the hell is the doctor? The wait must mean something is wrong.* I abandon my effort to think positive. *If there weren't a problem, we'd be out the door by now.* My stomach churns and keeps me on edge. Susan dozes off, then wakes up in no condition to indicate any concern.

The needle is stuck on the record playing in my brain, a vinyl record. My mind seeks a dark place: the surgeon is garnering the courage to tell us the unwelcome news. I get so worked up over what seems like an eternity that I barely recognize Dr. Happy as he struts through the jumble of white-coated nurses and doctors at the far, far end of the room. Susan spots him first.

"Sam, here he comes."

"Good news!" he blurts out, almost shouting. "It's just plain old scar tissue from the previous biopsy. That's what your doctor felt! Don't worry! No tumor, no cancer, I'm sure of it! Of course, we need to get a copy of the lab report, but I'm not concerned in the least. It's just plain old scar tissue!"

It feels as if the entire room hears him and is about to break out in wild applause. Instead, it's just me. I don't realize just how worried I've been until I almost cry with joy. I turn around to look at Susan, desperately wanting to hug her. I can't with that damned IV sticking out of her right arm. My anxious sense of something gone very wrong disappears. I hear "just plain old scar tissue" and want to believe the words. Maybe everything is going to be okay. Maybe. Always "maybe" with me.

The exit routine is familiar. A nurse brings Susan down to the entrance while I run down to get the car out of the underground parking garage. I pull up to the door. Susan, still slightly loopy, is rolled out and helped by the nurse into the vehicle.

By the time we get home, Susan mumbles words about how great everything turned out and nods off to sleep as soon as I tuck her into bed. I head to the office for an afternoon of work. My executive assistant, Eleanor, now a close and loving friend, is not happy about Susan at home in bed by herself.

Susan had been so sure from the start that the biopsy would not be cancer that she insisted we not tell anyone about the procedure. Not even our kids. So, we don't have to make phone calls to let everyone know the results. After all, in the year 2000, most people still don't have email or texting; heck, they don't even have cell phones.

Three days later, at eight in the morning, the telephone rings.

I have one foot out that door to the garage heading to work, but I pause. A bit early for a telephone call. Susan answers. "Yes, this is she," she says.

Susan waves me back into the house. "One moment, please." She holds the receiver up to her chest: "It's Dr. Morgan's office. The lab report is back. They want both of us to come in tomorrow to talk to Dr. Morgan. Can you do it? 10:30 a.m."

I nod my head in the affirmative. Susan confirms the appointment and hangs up. I'll clear my calendar for tomorrow morning when I get to the office. Eleanor will take care of rescheduling any appointments.

Susan gives me a sort of thumbs-up, a we're-set-for-tomorrow gesture as if nothing has happened, and I head to the garage. I sit in the car for a second and take several long, slow breaths, sensing that something is wrong. *What is it about me?* I think to myself. *Why can't I be like Susan?* Still, I wonder why she doesn't perceive this as bad news.

We arrive fifteen minutes early and expect the nurse to take us back to Dr. Morgan's, aka Dr. Happy's, office. Instead, he suddenly walks into the reception area to greet us. I notice he has an 8 ½ by 11-inch lined yellow writing pad in his right hand. A glance reveals a sketch of some sort on the top sheet. I also see that he's not smiling. Today's demeanor is entirely different than in our previous meetings.

He leads us into a narrow hallway flanked with one treatment door after another. "Let's see where we can find a place to talk," he says, poking his head into different rooms. Eventually, he announces, "This will do." He enters first into what at first seems like a closet. The long and narrow room can barely fit three people. He tosses his yellow pad on a small desk formed by an extended protrusion from the wall. He gestures for us to sit down.

As we all get settled, I look down at the yellow pad he placed on that small protrusion. I notice that the crude hand-drawn sketch on the top page is a doodle. The oxygen escapes the room. That sense of something wrong now scrapes my soul.

Not much conversation at first, just an awkward quiet with awkward motions. A scooting of chairs. The silence screams.

Suddenly, I find myself hovering above the scene as it unfolds below me.

I've had an out-of-body experience only once before, as a six-year-old having my tonsils out, also in a small room in the doctor's office. That's how they did that back in 1951. I had put on a tiny robe, climbed onto what seemed like an ironing board, and laid down. They put an ether mask over my mouth and asked me to breathe in and count backward from ten. "Ten, nnniiiine....." and I was out, except not really.

Instead, I was floating above the scene, my back almost touching the ceiling, looking down, and seeing myself on that ironing board as the doctors talked about me and worked on me. At least that was my dream.

Today, though, I am not wearing an ether mask, I am not being operated on, and I am not dreaming, though I wish I were. I can see myself seated at the rounded end of the small desk protrusion, along with that 8 ½ by 11 lined yellow pad, which Doctor Happy had been holding. Looking down from above, I magically reach down and pick it up. The sketch is hand-drawn.

Sloppy, I think. *Why isn't there a more professional presentation?*

I see crude, hand-drawn lines in the shape of a breast, small x's and dots at the top, and a shaded area at the bottom where the surgeon removed the tissue for testing.

Something new starts to happen, and I do not know what it is. A premonition? I think I hear something. A sound?

No. It is not a sound, maybe an image or hallucination? I don't understand. *Am I out-of-body; what the hell is going on?*

I wonder if, as Dr. Happy begins to talk, the universe notices that it might be time for an orchestra to form. Is it possible that I—Samuel Alan Simon, the husband of Susan for thirty-three of my fifty-four years, her first lover—and she—my first and only love—might have noticed that an orchestra has been called to form.

The only thing I do know is that something is terribly, terribly wrong, and the depth of that wrongness extends beyond the here and now, into the eternal, the stuff of primordial creation. At the precise instant that the doctor begins to talk, all the unknowable parts of the unknowable and unseeable universe shift and change and somehow let me know that everything—every single thing—is now different.

The doctor's voice breaks the spell. I am back, staring at the yellow pad in the center of the small desk. Neither Susan nor Dr. Happy has noticed my absence from the desk, looking down from above. Why would they, since I could see myself from above looking down as I sat in this very same seat?

"Stage 3," Dr. Happy says.

His words are strange. A new vocabulary I don't fully understand, though the meaning becomes clear.

"Why Stage 3?" I ask.

Susan sits to my right, facing Dr. Happy, silent, calm.

"Well, because of the size of the tissue with cancer and because we see no margins."

Jargon to me. "What are margins, Doc?" I'm frustrated, my tone more insistent than before.

"Well, remember, we didn't find a tumor. We just removed some breast tissue. A margin would have been where the breast cancer ended, and normal, healthy breast tissue began. I'm afraid that we found no normal breast tissue in what we took out of Susan. Just cancer."

Then we get more unwelcome news, delivered in Doctor Happy's calm, direct manner, using that same reassuring voice. "Well, let me describe the two types of breast cancer. One is known as *in situ*, where cancer sits, if you will, inside the breast ducts but has not invaded the tissue surrounding the ducts. It's called ductal carcinoma or DCIS in the medical world. The other type of breast cancer is called *invasive* or *infiltrating*. Here, cancer has invaded the tissue surrounding the ducts. Breast cancer is usually one or the other. Susan, I am afraid, has both".

Susan's breast cancer is not merely Stage 3. She has all three markers: The amount of tissue with cancer, the absence of margins, and both kinds of breast cancer. Any of these factors would warrant the classification Stage 3. Not good. Stage 3 cubed.

I know what the doctor's words mean. Susan's mother, Bertha (née Levy) Kalmans died at fifty-six from metastasized breast cancer. Susan is fifty-four.

CHAPTER 2

I Know How This Story Is Going to End

Susan's mom. I was there thirty-two years ago, on August 5th, 1967, the day she passed away from her Stage 4 breast cancer, just three weeks before our first wedding anniversary.

The breast cancer had metastasized and spread by the time we married on August 23rd, 1966. Indeed, Susan and I both suspect it was her mom's breast cancer that persuaded Susan's parents to agree to let us get married.

So, we move to Houston for the summer after college graduation to be with her mom as her breast cancer advances. She has gone from a robust woman with a personality that dominated the family to a thin, fragile frame. We all know the outcome, just not when.

On August 3rd, the doctor admits Susan's mom to the hospital. Bernice, Susan's oldest sister, is called up from

Brownsville, Texas, where she lives, to join us and Susan's two brothers as the vigil starts. A family member always sits in her room. When it is Susan's turn, she grabs my hand and guides me into the room with her.

The small hospital room, located at a distance from the nurse's station, is silent—no TV or radio playing— and dark since, as usual, the blinds remain down and shut. Pillows prop up Mom so she can see people. She smiles at me and whispers hello. Susan walks up next to her, straightens her hair, gives her some water to sip, and then sits down next to her. I take a seat in a chair that, oddly, is as far away as I can get.

On the morning of August 5th, the Kalmans' house receives an urgent call. Everyone needs to get to the hospital as soon as possible. The moment has arrived.

Susan and I rush over to the family home on Harvest Lane from our apartment to meet Susan's family. We all head over to the hospital together. Everyone is dower, focused, and in a rush. The business of death is unpleasant and urgent.

We ride up the large hospital elevator together. The elevator door opens onto the cancer floor, and we all beeline in the direction of Susan's mother's room. As we cross in front of the nurse's station, Buddy and his dad stop, look at me, and say, "Sam, why don't you stay out here?" Susan and I exchange glances. She doesn't protest, so neither do I. I face the nurse's station as they head off toward the room. I am still standing around when Melvin arrives after parking the car. He looks at me, and I point down to the right. He heads off without a word.

Susan's father and the four children—Bernice, Melvin, Buddy, and Susan—are in their mom's hospital room along with Melvin's wife, Roz, and Buddy's wife, Doris. I am too new, I guess, not yet melded into the fabric of their family. I wonder if I should ask or even insist on being with Susan at this moment. Instead, I just sit down in the waiting room. Not an intimate family waiting room. Not the waiting room near the hospital room where the family has gathered. The big waiting room for the entire floor, with hallways off to the right and the left.

I feel empty and alone sitting by myself in this sizable waiting area outside the nurse's station. No one is near me because everyone else seems to have somewhere to go or be. The nurses are busy at their stations. They don't notice me. I feel as if I am invisible. I turn deep inside of myself, looking for clarity, yet I only experience confusion.

I wonder if I am supposed to feel something related to Susan's mom, but instead, I just feel alone and sad. Terribly alone. I wish someone were here to hold me and wonder why I was being left alone out here to cry. The nurses do not notice. No one walks over to comfort me.

Time stands still for me. Despite the relentless intercom and the intermittent beeping of whirring machines, a silence aches within me. A hollowness. I look around through the tears in my eyes. Mouths are moving. Phones must be ringing because I see nurses pick up the receiver. It is as if I am not even here—that I am somewhere else.

The wait ends as the men appear from the hallway to my right. Susan and Bernice, Roz, and Doris follow behind. I sit up straight, wipe my eyes. *What if they notice I cried?*

The group pauses briefly to pick me up, then moves with purpose toward the exit. Melvin says he will get the car and bring it around. Buddy heads to the payphones. "I need to make some calls now," he tells the air as he pulls out a list of names and numbers. Buddy and his wife, Doris, drove separately from the rest of us, and will meet us back at the house after Buddy makes his calls.

Susan, pale and quiet, looks straight at me, a blank stare, then grabs my arm and puts her forehead on my shoulder. She begins to shake as she quietly sobs. I hold her tight. It breaks my heart, yet I am so grateful that I can be here with her at this moment.

Back at the Harvest Lane home where Susan grew up, the living room fills slowly with family and neighbors. The religious practices committee of Beth Yeshurun, the conservative Jewish congregation where Susan's family has belonged for generations, requires burial within twenty-four hours of death whenever possible. Planning needs to start now!

Today, thirty-three years later, sitting in this narrow, closet-like room, I translate Doctor Happy's "Stage 3" pronouncement into "Stage 3 cubed," and I know, in the deepest part of my soul—I know what that means.

I don't say anything. I don't run around crying and telling people Susan is about to die. Of course, the response would be, "Oh Sam, don't be silly. She's strong. Medicine has changed radically in these past thirty-three years." So, I don't say it out loud to anyone, ever.

I also see a parallel in what happened to Susan's mother and how we, Susan and I, have handled Susan's breast care. Maybe it is our fault. Susan's mother waited almost two years before getting the lump in her breast examined. Susan's grandmother, her father's mother, Rose Lewis Kalmans, who lived with the Harvest Lane family, had suffered a heart attack two years earlier. Susan's mom felt the lump during a self-examination yet insisted on waiting until Grandma Rosie recovered before dealing with her health issues.

Now, it is us, Susan and I, who have delayed. We have waited five years since a clarion signal that something is wrong inside her breast. We didn't see it, though now I wonder if we were blind to the obvious.

First, it was insane to wait thirteen years before we even started to monitor Susan's breast. No one back then recommended mammograms for women in their twenties and early thirties, yet Susan's mom had died from breast cancer.

Susan's first routine medical breast exam came in the mid-1980s. The following two exams provoked a needle biopsy of what then seemed like a lump. Both biopsies turned out normal.

Susan's third biopsy should have screamed at us, yet we ignored it. Her annual mammogram in 1995 concerned the radiologist. It showed an area that looked different from the rest of the breast. It didn't seem to be a lump, just a site that looked dark. It could have been anything. We have since learned, again, something we should have discovered back then, that Susan has "dense breasts," which can make it hard to know what the dark areas on a mammogram mean. The next step was a biopsy. Susan had changed internists since the last biopsy, and he referred her to a new breast surgeon.

At the first appointment, the breast surgeon explained that protocols have evolved since her last biopsy fifteen years before. He would remove some tissue from the area that looks suspicious, and the lab technicians in the operating room would perform what they called a "frozen section." The tissue would be flash-frozen and examined under powerful microscopes by the technicians. If the tissue tested normal, Susan would get up, get dressed, and we would go home. If the tissue tested positive for cancer, the standard of care called for the surgeon to remove the breast.

I carefully researched this new approach and checked it out. Even though Ralph Nader, the famous consumer crusader, my first boss, had decided to run for president, he still took my call. He didn't support the approach and suggested I check with his health expert, Sid Wolfe. Both Ralph and Sid recommended we take a different route, and

Susan and I agreed. We told the surgeon that no matter the breast tissue test results in the operating room, we wanted to get a second opinion before deciding on surgery. We did not want any treatment until we were confident in the diagnosis. We were aware of the possibility of false negatives and no false-positive results from these quick in-the-room tests.

The discussion with the breast surgeon was not easy. Persuading any doctor to do things differently is never easy, and in this situation, it was no small matter. Indeed, despite the clarity of our request, the doctor came out of the surgical area, surgical gown and cap and mask still on, to try to persuade me otherwise. "Sam, it looks like cancer. You should approve a mastectomy, especially given her family history. Susan said to ask you, and she will do whatever you decide."

It took all my strength to say, "No, we discussed this. We need to make sure, and we want the second opinion."

He reluctantly agreed. The tissue was sent to a nearby lab at Inova Fairfax hospital for their opinion. It turned out to be a bit of a mystery even for them. Inova wasn't sure, so they sent the sample to Mayo Clinic for a third opinion. Mayo's response was simply that the tissue was "extremely interesting," and they wanted someone to keep them informed, whatever that meant.

The doctor handed us a copy of the report from Mayo to take with us. Mayo, Inova, Susan's surgeon, and internist all told us to follow Susan's breast very closely.

Instead of hearing a blaring siren or seeing a swirling red light telling us to head back to the hospital and get that mastectomy, we simply filed the report away and got on with our lives. In retrospect, that seems to have been the functional equivalent of Susan's mother deciding to wait two years to have a doctor examine her lump.

Now, in the Spring of 2000, sitting in Dr. Happy's closet-like room, I know how the story is going to end. I am nauseous at the prospect of accompanying Susan through her end-of-days. I don't know if I can do it.

Susan? How does Susan feel about all of this? Honestly, I'm not sure. We seem to exist on separate planes of the universe. She doesn't act as if the universe has shifted or changed.

"You need a mastectomy," Dr. Happy tells her. She doesn't even react outwardly to this news.

I am the one who asks about the other, the left breast. No one can tell if any cancer is in the left breast because there wasn't even a tumor in the right breast; there was just cancer. We all agree—a double mastectomy. Doctor Happy wants to do it soon. He says we should begin to look for an oncologist.

We need to make some phone calls. The universe may know what has happened. Susan and I need to alert everyone else.

The first time I cry is later that afternoon. Inside, I am in a bit of an existential panic, though I work ridiculously hard not to show it to Susan, who seems calm, her usual self. Not sure what to do, yet feeling like we need to do something, we decide to call our temple, Temple Rodef Shalom, to let them know about Susan's Stage 3 cubed breast cancer. I ask to speak with the new, young rabbi. She is out of town, so we are put through to the temple cantor.

"Hello, Sam," I hear, and as I try to respond, I choke up, start to cry. I hand the phone to Susan.

"Michael, it's Susan," she says in a dry, matter-of-fact tone. "Sorry about that. We want you to know that I have been diagnosed with breast cancer and that I will be having a double mastectomy as soon as the doctor can schedule it." Just like that. Calm and confident.

Susan puts us on speakerphone, and the cantor asks us both, "Can I put Susan's name on the *Misheberach* list?"

The tradition in our reform Jewish congregation is for the rabbi to read aloud at *Kabbalat Shabbat,* Friday night services, the names of congregants who are ill. The congregation then chants a prayer asking God to heal both body and soul of those who require such healing. Susan's body and my soul both need healing, it seems. So that *Erev Shabbat,* Friday night, Susan and I sit in the same seats we have been sitting in every Friday night for the last twenty-seven years, listening to other names read aloud.

The rabbi reads the names during the service in the order in which they were added to the list, so she reads Susan's name aloud last: "…and Susan Simon."

We close our eyes, squeeze our hands tighter, and chant with the congregation the *Misheberach* prayer.

Misheberach imoteinu
M'kor habrachah l'avoteinu
Bless those in need of healing with r'fuah sh'lemah
The renewal of body,
The Renewal of Spirit
And let us say
Amen

When the chanting stops, stillness fills the sanctuary. The cantor sings the "amen" in a way that lingers in the air: "Ahhh, Ahhh, Ahhh Ahh-men." We keep our eyes shut for a few seconds and squeeze our hands even tighter. My eyes tear up. Susan is stoic.

A reception called an *Oneg Shabbat* follows the service in the social hall. We walk out of the sanctuary to the adjoining room. We call it the "social hall." Immediately, Susan's friends rush up to her and ask, each in their unique way: "Why is your name on the list, Susan?"

Susan quietly tells them. I stand back and watch, not wanting to intrude on what seems private space for each of these seemingly intimate conversations.

After the crowd of people who have come to check on Susan thins, her friend Sharon approaches slowly with what at first seems like a glare. "What did you not tell me, girl?"

Susan, who is the taller of the two, bends down, puts her hands on Sharon's shoulder and her forehead on Sharon's. I hear the words as they lock their eyes together. "Breast cancer," Susan says softly.

My eyes tear up as I expect Susan now, finally, to break down and cry. Maybe even collapse. Instead, I am the one who senses at this moment, not a beginning but an ending—an inevitable step in a predestined journey.

Once again, with Susan and her friend Sharon forehead-to-forehead, seemingly frozen together at that moment, I am desperately alone in a room full of people, experiencing the events that take place beyond my control. Tears roll down my cheeks. I look around to make sure no one is noticing.

I shake myself out of this moment, feeling self-indulgent. *What the hell is wrong with you, Sam?" I lecture myself. "You are not the one with breast cancer. You do know that.* I don't feel sorry for myself. It just seems that I am the only one who knows how this story is going to end.

CHAPTER 3

The Story of Susan and Sam

This story, Susan and Sam's story, begins on an afternoon in December of 1961, about forty years before the fateful moment in the office of Doctor Morgan (aka Dr. Happy). I am one of two sixteen-year-old boys sitting on stage in the Hilton Hotel's ballroom in Texarkana, Texas. We are the candidates running to be regional *Mazkir* (Hebrew for secretary) of the Texoma Region of B'nai B'rith Youth Organization.

On stage now, I scan the folks in the ballroom and notice this curly-haired girl, with big braces on her teeth, staring up at me. Like directly at me. I stare back for a second and note her smile. She's cute, but I can't focus on that now. I continue the scan, trying to feel the energy, judge the room.

No surprise, I lose. El Paso cannot compete against the big cities in the region, like Houston, Dallas, Oklahoma City, San Antonio. They each have large delegations, with more than half of the people coming from Houston and

Dallas. El Paso's delegation is almost always too small for one of us to win anything. Still, I try. After my concession speech, in which I lecture everyone on how unfair this situation is to El Paso kids, I receive a standing ovation.

"You should have given that speech first," says someone I've never met.

As the room empties, I look around for the girl with curly black hair staring at me earlier. I urgently poke my head up (I'm six feet tall already) and scan the room. I see her across the way, heading toward the exit with friends. She pauses, turns around, and looks toward me! Our eyes meet for a moment. The girl next to her tugs at her to keep moving out of the room. She glances back and smiles. In a hotel ballroom filled with hundreds of us teenagers, what is it about her that catches my attention? Why the smile? Is it meant for me?

That girl turns out to be Susan Meryl Kalmans, from Houston. In the convention's waning moments, I look out for her, always noticing her in that sixteen-year-old boy sort of way. I never do get up the guts to introduce myself.

The following day, I board a Greyhound bus waiting in the hotel parking lot with the sign "Dallas." I travel to Dallas with the convention group, then take a regular Greyhound back to El Paso. I sit next to a window and stare at all the other kids searching for their bus, a few cars with parents packing up small groups. As the bus pulls away and crawls through the narrow parking lot lanes, I notice her—the girl with curly black hair and big braces—walking alongside the bus on the sidewalk. She is waving like crazy. Big smile! I stare. *Is she waving at me?* I wonder. Many years later, she tells me she *was* waving at me. Really.

Amazingly, three short years later, that curly-haired girl shows up in El Paso as a member of the 1963 freshman class of Texas Western College (TWC). TWC is the only local, four-year college in El Paso, which most local high school graduates attend. Out-of-town students are rare, with the female ones always stirring the interest of us local fellows.

Susan and my journey are almost diametrically opposite. Susan ends up at TWC because it is the farthest she can get from Houston and stay in Texas. Her family agrees because a cousin lives in El Paso. The Army has stationed her older brother Buddy in El Paso for a year. I am at Texas Western for two reasons—my high school grades are not that good, and my family can't afford for me to live away from home. They say I need to earn a scholarship if I want to go away from El Paso to college. My goal, then, is to get good grades and save money so I can transfer to the University of Texas in Austin after two years at TWC. That's what my oldest sister Marion did.

My one diversion is the Jewish fraternity known as Sammy or Sigma Alpha Mu (ΣAM). At one of the first "mixers"—just a party with ΣAM and the Jewish sorority Alpha Epsilon Phi (AEPhi)—I am introduced to Susan Meryl Kalmans. She smiles and says I look familiar. I think she does, too, though I don't remember from where. This Susan doesn't have braces, and her hair isn't that curly. (I later learn she and her friends iron each other's hair straight.) I am very interested. Unfortunately, she's already with someone, Mike Bernstein. Mike is a nerdy, dull, numbers kind of guy with a pen holder in his shirt pocket. He is older, a junior dating a freshman. They are not going steady as far as I can tell.

As I suspected, that relationship doesn't last, but Susan starts to date another guy before I can raise my hand. Steve is from New York and a smoother talker—the opposite of Mike.

I need to figure out a way to spend time with Susan. I have a go-to friend and date, Jane, a freshman who grew up with me in El Paso. I suggest to Steve that he and Susan go out one night with the two of us. Neither Jane nor Steve is aware of my ulterior motive to reconnect with Susan.

We end up at the dog races in Juarez, Mexico. The dog track is a bit of a drive once we cross the border to Mexico in downtown El Paso.

I like the long drive and take every opportunity to talk with Susan. In the stands at the track, I sit between the two women with Steve on the outside. Of course, Jane is bored silly since I ignore her to speak with Susan, and Steve is interested in the dogs. He delights in throwing $3 on every race, which was a lot of money back then. The most fun for me and the two girls is to hear the voice over the loudspeaker at the start of each race announce, "And here comes the bunny!"

Neither of our dates is going that well, so we leave early. Since Steve drove, I suggest that Susan and I sit in the back and Jane in the front with Steve. Steve and Jane shrug their shoulders. "Okay, whatever," they agree.

Yes! Our first date! Okay, maybe a half-date or sort-of-date.

I jump into the back seat of the car and get as close to Susan as possible. I can't tell if she thinks I'm just crude or interested. I tell her she looks familiar, and I ask her about that Texoma convention. She is coy and says it might have been her. Back on campus, it is evident that I want to start dating. Now. I am impulsive and impatient, while Susan is stoic, patient, and cautious. I ask her out.

"I can't, Sam, I'm with Steve, and we agreed not to date other people."

I test her. "Steve doesn't have to know." She just shakes her head, reinforcing her "no."

Susan plans to spend the summer after our freshman school year in Houston. Steve is staying in El Paso to go to summer school. I have a job at the local haberdashery, Al's Shop for Men, selling men's clothing. I am working to earn and save enough money to go away to school after the sophomore year. With the drama of my pursuit of Susan on hold, I call Jane for a movie date. "I can't, Sam," she tells me. "Steve and I are going out for dinner. We've been hanging out recently."

As soon as I hang up, I call Susan in Houston. "Susan, Jane just told me she has a date with Steve tomorrow night, and this is not the first time they've gone out. Can we date now?"

She remains cool and calm as if nothing significant happened. No crying. No anger. Just, "Let me see what is going on when I get back, Sam." It drives me crazy.

I don't know what happens between Steve and Susan after she gets back from Houston, except when I call Susan to check in, she tells me that she and Steve have broken up. I ask her out, and on October 4th, 1964, Susan and I have our first official date.

We go to a movie, followed by a snack at the Mesa Motel coffee shop near my home. And we talk. Susan finally confirms that it was her at the convention, and she does remember me and the election. She also confesses that she sort of chased the bus that day. I learn much more about her family, her life in Houston, her Judaism. I tell her all about my family. We note that both her father and my father work in the clothing business. And so do I! Susan mirrors my enthusiasm.

It doesn't take us long to find our way to the romantic places in El Paso—the Scenic Drive car park and the Rim Road overlook—the usual spots where folks "parked" for romantic times (and deeds). Six weeks go by, and we agree not to date other people. In high school, we would have said we were "going steady." In the college fraternity and sorority worlds, formal rituals mark the decision to be exclusive and enshrine these commitments. First is the practice of becoming "dropped." The fraternity man gives a necklace to his girlfriend with the Greek Letters of the fraternity, in this case, ΣAM, who then wears it to alert all the other guys that she's taken. Susan is "dropped" by Sam on November 28th, 1964. We are a thing. We are going steady.

At nineteen years old, our relationship is on fire. Hot, hot, hot! We can't seem to get enough of each other. I tell my parents about Susan, and she becomes a familiar fixture in our house. We often head to my home to study in the living room in the evenings at a bridge table. My parents enjoy Susan and are delighted that she is Jewish. Being Jewish is the most important thing about this relationship for both our families.

We spend all our free time together. We study together, eat together, hang out with the same friends, and go to all the fraternity and sorority events together. Especially basketball games. The Texas Western Basketball Team, the "Miners," are nationally ranked. They are playing in the NCAA finals; by the time we graduate, the team will be crowned national champions.

A group of Susan's friends conspires with us to let Susan stay out later than the 9 p.m. dorm curfew. Susan can call one of them, who will stand ready to open an emergency-exit side door to the women's dorm when she knocks. She routinely sneaks back in at 10 or 11 p.m. or even later.

Infatuated and in love, we are ready for the next step. We move from "being dropped" to "getting pinned." In these exotic rituals of the Greek (even Jewish Greek) fraternity and sorority systems, getting "pinned" is a signal of the intent to get married and includes a pre-engagement ceremony during which I must ask Susan to accept the fraternity pin. After taking off the necklace, I will pin the small, circular black stone with gold Greek letters ΣAM onto her blouse. On February 27th, exactly two months after getting "dropped," I attach the pin. We are now officially "pinned."

Susan's parents, who sense this is getting serious, now want to meet me. We arrange for the long drive to Houston and back during the spring vacation of 1964. It is the first of what will be many cross-state car trips that usually take thirteen hours each way.

I've never been to Houston. As we hit the outskirts at approximately nine in the evening, Susan starts giving me the turn-by-turn directions. She tells me about the parts of town where her parents once owned a clothing store and the house we are going to on the other side of town. We pull into the driveway around 10 p.m.

The home is located in a quaint, quiet neighborhood a few blocks from the University of Houston's (U of H) main campus. Neighbors are middle-class folks, ranging from professors at the U of H to salesmen like Susan's dad. My work at Al's Shop for Men will stand me in good stead with the family. Since selling their clothing store, her Dad, Joe Kalmans, has worked in the Sakowitz department store's men's department. Her uncle, Sam Kalmans, is a regional manager for Bond Department Store on Main street in downtown Houston. He hires me to work in their menswear section to help cover employees taking summer vacations.

Susan's family graciously welcomes me into their home. Grandma Rosie is my favorite. I love her! She is a pistol—short, sharp, and still smokes, even after her heart attack. Yes! I can smoke too.

I get an intense interrogation about who I am, my family, and my Jewish background and practice. Susan's

Dad especially wants to know what I intend to do in life. Both of her older brothers are graduates of Texas A&M University and are engineers, working at different Houston businesses. Susan's oldest sibling—a sister sixteen years her senior—was married at twenty-three, considered old back then, to Ruben Edelstein. His family owns a chain of furniture stores in Brownsville and McAllen, Texas, also known as The Valley. I need to measure up to all of that, it seems.

I also need to be on good behavior. "Your bedroom is the first room to the right at the top of the stairs," Susan's folks specify when it's time to settle in. The room had been Grandma Rosie's until her heart attack not that long ago, at which point the family remodeled to put a bedroom and bathroom downstairs so she would not have to climb up to the second floor. Susan sleeps in what used to be her bedroom growing up, which is at the opposite end of the hall from where I will sleep. I fantasize about us getting together there one night. There is something erotic about having sex with Susan in the bedroom where she grew up. Instead, she introduces me to Hermann Park and its duck pond. A place for young couples to go for just those sorts of activities. The euphemism "let's go watch the ducks" survives to this day.

Our passion for each other masks the undertone of a much bigger issue in the Kalmans family. We are not noticing or hearing the concern about Susan's mother. Perhaps the family doesn't want to burden us with the news.

Susan's mother has been diagnosed with breast cancer. The decision by Susan's mother to delay any evaluation of the lump on her breast until things with Grandma Rosie settled will turn out to be a tragic mistake. The lump is cancer, and she will have a double mastectomy in the coming months.

As Susan and I drive back to El Paso, we talk about her mother. Susan is adamant that she be with her mother for the treatment. I cannot imagine being apart from Susan for the entire summer. I need to figure out how to be in Houston for the summer of 1965.

As soon as we get back and settled in El Paso, we call Susan's Uncle Sam Kalmans, the regional manager for the Bond Department Store in Houston, about a possible job for me over the coming summer. Susan's father, Joe Kalmans, is a bit of a gruff, everyday sort of guy. Uncle Sam, his brother, is a smooth corporate executive who has spent much of his adult life in California. Uncle Sam is delighted to find a summer job for his niece's boyfriend. I am a backup for the full-time staff as they take their summer vacations. My parents understand and reassure me this is the right move.

Once in Houston, it doesn't take us long to settle into a routine. I quickly find an apartment with a roommate near Susan's home. I spend my time during the day working at the Bond Department Store and with Susan and her family at their home in the evenings.

Susan's mother enters treatment for her breast cancer and has that double mastectomy. During a visit to the hospital, Susan and her older brother Melvin, her sibling closest in age, learn that their mom's breast cancer has metastasized throughout the rest of her body. She will need immediate and aggressive chemotherapy and radiation treatments. Her prognosis is highly uncertain.

I fear Susan will collapse into an emotional puddle at the prospect of her mother's death. I can almost hear her next words in my head: "I've got to be here for her. I am sorry, Sam, but I need to transfer to the University of Houston." What would I do if that happens? Maybe I can transfer too?

Susan surprises me with her composure. So does her mom. "Don't worry, we will be fine," her mom insists when Susan says she is thinking of staying in Houston. "Live your lives; don't worry about me." Susan does not transfer.

The rest of the summer flies by in a blur of work and summer backyard BBQs at Susan's home. Her dad grills. Susan and I fit in with the rest of the family. We belong here. We are just like her siblings and their wives—a solid couple in the family, or so it seems. The next step is obvious, almost a technicality.

At the end of the summer, we both go back to El Paso with a new mission. We are in love, and we want to get married. Now! While Susan's mom is still around.

Across the vast expanse of Texas from El Paso to Houston, it becomes apparent that our parents do not mirror our enthusiasm. When I talk to my parents, I get, "Take it slow, Sam. You're too young. You have a full life ahead of you." Susan receives the same signals from hers.

"Wait awhile, Dear," our parents say. "Date some other girls (boys); if what you feel is true love, you two will get back together again."

During the fall of 1965, Susan's mother's condition continues to worsen. She is not going to survive her breast cancer. As a result, both sets of parents relent and grant their blessing for our marriage. Neither family wants to get in the way of Susan's mother participating in her youngest daughter's wedding.

Urgent questions now need to be answered: Where are we going to live? What am I going to do with my life?

I signed up for ROTC my freshman year at my parents' insistence. My sister Evelyn was already married to a West Point graduate, now a lieutenant in the Army. Given my poor high school grades, there was a sense I might not do that well in college. They viewed the military as a safe career. They remember the Great Depression. Plus, being an officer has honor in their eyes compared to an enlisted grunt. As an officer, I could retire in twenty years with a good government pension. At the end of my sophomore year, I apply for and win one of the first-ever U.S. Army ROTC full-tuition college scholarships. The U.S. Army will pay for one hundred percent of my college expenses anywhere I want to go in the United States, as long as they have an ROTC program. We can now go to Austin for the junior and senior years, with all my college expenses paid!

My grades are excellent, a 3.8 grade point average, so getting a transfer shouldn't be a problem for me. Susan's grades, however, are not, and she might not be able to transfer. Plus, her family is in the middle of a crisis. I am in love with Susan, so I am not about to go without her, period, end of discussion. We will stay at Texas Western here in El Paso. We are already a couple, and we prefer to get married than transfer schools.

So how do we get married? We are not even twenty years old yet. At one point, we briefly consider eloping to Juarez, Mexico, which, of course, would upset our families even more than marrying at this young age. Besides, the impetus for the rush to get married is for Susan's mom to be in attendance, and sneaking off to Juarez will just make things worse.

There are more questions. We don't even know how we can afford married life. Susan plans to be a teacher, but I need to figure out what I want to do with my life.

My passion is politics and government, with a focus on fairness and justice. I want to help the "little guy." I am already a veteran crusader in the community. At fourteen years old, I started a petition drive in El Paso against a proposed 11 p.m. curfew for anyone under seventeen years of age. I believed the city was unfairly targeting the Mexican kids in the ghettos of El Paso. In college, I am active in the Student Senate. I tend to argue with everyone about everything. While I fret over what I should do in life, it seems that all my friends know that I am a natural for law school. I apply to the University of Texas School of Law in Austin.

Another and perhaps more important reason to go to graduate school in 1967, the year of my expected graduation, is that the Vietnam War is now raging. The war is highly controversial and not going very well. The press is filled with stories about troops losing confidence in brand new commanders and killing the new second lieutenants not long after they arrive in Vietnam. These fragging events escalate to the point that the Army cannot get new lieutenants—referred to as cannon fodder in newspaper articles—trained and sent to Vietnam fast enough.

Vietnam wasn't on the horizon when I signed up for ROTC as a freshman, nor the following year when I took the scholarship. I regret having accepted the money for many reasons, but especially when I learn that scholarship students are considered the elite in ROTC. We are required to serve in what is known as a combat arms division. When I get assigned to the infantry, it feels like my success will turn out to be a death sentence.

I apply for a deferment so I can go to law school. Not only do I like to argue, I think that maybe by my graduation in 1970, the future will also be brighter. The deferment should be a routine matter. My PMS, Professor of Military Studies, a young Army captain, assured me before I even applied that the scholarship would not interfere with me going to graduate school, whether law school or any other program.

A plan is coming together. We discover that Susan can graduate early—in August 1966 rather than May

1967—by doing her practice teaching and taking a giant class load in the spring semester of 1966. If she attends both summer sessions in 1966, she could have a job teaching by the fall. We just need to sell Susan's school counselor and convince both our families.

Okay, here is the plan: The Army grants my deferment, I get accepted to law school, Susan's counselor agrees to her early graduation, and both sets of parents agree to our plan. Waiting for calls and approvals becomes the story of our short lives as a couple.

Now, gulp, I need to phone Susan's father and ask him for his daughter's hand in marriage.

Susan calls me silly and old-fashioned. "You do not need to call my father to ask permission to marry me! He knows we're getting married. It's no secret." Her reluctance makes me wonder if she knows something I don't know. Maybe she has heard some talk at home. She even asks me what I plan to say or do if her dad says no.

"Oh, come on, Susan, asking your father is just a formality. I make the call. "Mr. Kalmans (I don't call him Joe), I love Susan. I would like your permission to marry your daughter. I love Susan and want her to be my wife." The conversation is short and awkward. I know he can tell that I'm nervous. He wants to know what I intend to do with my life and how I plan to support his daughter. I tell him I am going to become a lawyer. I also reassure him that I will be an Army officer first and that this is a very secure job.

I hear a reluctant yes. I will feel this same hesitancy or skepticism I initially experienced this first summer for years to come. Maybe no man is good enough for a father's youngest daughter, or perhaps he is consumed by his wife, Susan's mother's, breast cancer.

When we call Susan's siblings to share our good news, we hear something new from her brothers, Melvin and Buddy. "You should plan your wedding soon," they both indicate. "Mom isn't doing well."

We tell my parents, and they call and talk to Susan's parents. The four will be what in Yiddish is called *Mishpucha*, which means non-blood-related family. A pleasant call. My dad and Susan's dad are both clothing (*shmattah* in Yiddish) salesmen, so they have a lot in common.

The telephone calls start flying between the two sets of parents and siblings as we try to nail down logistics. Everyone has an idea. Who can be there and who cannot on what date? Etc., etc. A plan built around speed and practicality eventually comes together, and we all agree on August 23rd, 1966, for the wedding date. The Kalmans want to throw an engagement party and announce the wedding in January of 1966.

One more thing. I still need to propose to Susan formally. I don't have a wedding ring, and I don't have any money. I worry about my folks wagging their fingers, lecturing me: "We told you to wait!"

Instead, my mom lovingly explains the basics of wedding rings. First is the engagement ring, which usually has a diamond. There is then a matching wedding band that generally doesn't have a diamond. I listen and act as if I knew all this, which of course, I did not. I hadn't even thought about rings.

She takes me to a local jewelry store where she knows the manager to select a ring and a wedding band set. She will put them on layaway, which is how credit is granted in these times before credit cards become universal. Together, we pick out a silver, one-carat diamond ring with a minor, barely noticeable flaw and a plain connecting wedding band. We put them on layaway with a $100 down payment that Mom lends me; I will pay the rest of the $600 price tag directly to the store with what I earn at my job at Al's Shop for Men.

I decided to propose to Susan on the evening of the annual AEPhi sorority formal fall dance. Perfect time and place. Susan will be in a gown, and I'll be in a tuxedo. The venue is the Hilton Hotel at the El Paso International Airport.

I make the final payment and pick up the ring two days before the dance. At the first break for the band, I ask Susan to walk with me outside to the swimming pool area, ostensibly for me to smoke a cigarette. We feel the warm evening air and slight breeze as we exit the ballroom onto the swimming pool deck, which thankfully lies empty and silent. The pool lights seem to shine up toward the luminous moon. At this moment, there doesn't even seem to be a single airplane taking off or landing, or maybe I just don't hear the noise.

I invite Susan to sit down on a bench, then kneel. "Susan, I love you," I say softly. "Will you marry me?" The one real surprise tonight is the ring I pull out of my pocket and slip on her finger. The diamond looks enormous to us, two nineteen-year-old kids.

"Yes! Yes!" She jumps up and holds out her hand to stare at the one-carat diamond. I don't think I have ever seen her so beautiful than at this moment with her hand out front, fingers stretched apart, big smile. She turns away from the diamond and wraps herself around me with the biggest, deepest kiss ever. "Yes! I love you too." I wonder if we really know what love means, even at this moment.

She returns immediately to her calm and focused self. Taking my hand, she says: "Let's go tell everybody," and pulls me back to the ballroom just as the orchestra is making its way back onto the stage. "We just got engaged," one of us whispers to the band leader, and he invites us onto the stage.

"Please. May I have your attention?" the band leader says into the mic. "I'd like to present the future, Mr. & Mrs. Sam Simon." Susan holds out her hand with the diamond sparkling in the light. Everyone turns and applauds. I am on top of the world!

We dance the next dance with each other, then rush to a payphone to call both sets of parents to let them know. Sam Simon and Susan Kalmans are engaged.

Our life quickly becomes a blur. The urgency to move forward and get everything done reflects, in part, the ardent desire for Susan's mom to experience her daughter get married. In January of 1966, I fly to Houston with my parents for the engagement party. I am twenty years old and have never flown in an airplane. It scares me to death. When the wheels come down for landing, I think we are going to crash.

At the engagement party, Susan and I are the centers of attention. We love it. Houston's *Jewish Week* features an announcement along with Susan's picture.

Back in El Paso, Susan's class load is crushing. She is solid as always and gets it all done. Susan barely has the time to go home to see her mother at the end of May before starting summer school in June. In Houston, she experiences a new mother and calls me in tears to describe her. "It's awful, Sam. She has lost so much weight and now walks with a cane. I don't know if Mom will be able to walk down the aisle. Dad holds her by the arm so she doesn't fall. She's so frail. I can't believe how much she's changed."

Susan is almost sobbing as she talks about her mom, then she takes a breath and returns to the core Susan. I note how her focus and calm nature in the face of school pressure and her mother's failing health is a defining trait of the essential Susan. She is going to need to tap into that again and again.

Susan's mom knows her daughter and senses her anxiety. She doesn't want her condition to dominate the wedding nor the planning for the wedding. Much like Susan, she continues to command the stage despite her failing health, her inner strength very much intact. After all, her baby is getting married.

August 23rd, 1966, is the big day, but the wedding is not large by Houston Jewish standards. The ceremony takes place in the congregation's smallest venue, the Greenfield Chapel. The wedding reception and party will be in the synagogue's social hall, not a big downtown hotel. Susan's parents have invited immediate family and only their closest friends. We have only a handful of people coming from El Paso. The guests total around 150 people.

The day itself is chaotic for me. I wonder if all grooms feel the same at their wedding, a bystander in what might be the most crucial moment of their life. Or maybe it's because I just turned twenty-one years old. The wedding coordinator, a friend of Susan's family, greets my family as we enter the building and reassures us that everything will be just fine. I hope so, as I have never done this before.

This moment is just an extension of the last few days. I go along, doing whatever anyone tells me to, learning to say, "Yes, dear."

Indeed, everything falls into place as it should. Susan's brothers are my groomsmen and enter the chapel first. Next, my dad, who is the best man, and I walk down the aisle. The rabbi then comes in, followed by flower girls. The ceremony goes without a glitch until the rabbi turns to me and asks, "Do you, Sam Simon, take Susan Meryl Kalmans as your lawfully wedded wife?" The expected response is "I do." My answer: "Yes."

My response elicits a muted chuckle from the pews. "I now pronounce you husband and wife." I get to stomp on a light bulb wrapped in a decorated sleeve. Then, "Ladies and gentlemen, Mr. & Mrs. Samuel A. Simon."

Susan and I turn to each other. We both smile, and once again, those beautiful brown, sparkling eyes staring into my "bedroom eyes," and we kiss. And kiss, and the room starts chuckling again. I don't remember who put their hand on my shoulder to end it, but somebody did. Susan and I turn, straighten ourselves, and walk back down the aisle, arm in arm. Me, twenty-one years old, Susan twenty. What are we thinking?

What do we know? As is traditional in Jewish weddings, Susan and I are escorted to a private dressing area together for some "private time." Okay, nobody told us what to do alone in this room for about fifteen or twenty minutes, with Susan's brothers standing guard outside. It takes us a moment to figure it isn't about having sex but feeling the moment, the sacred moment, of being husband and wife. We are excited and pleased and have no frigging idea about life as a married couple.

Our honeymoon turns into an extended four-day drive from Houston to El Paso. Susan's teaching job starts three weeks earlier than we thought, so we cancel plans for a honeymoon in Mexico City. We missed the fine print that required new teachers to attend an extended training session; oops.

Instead, we arrange for a few nights in a cabin in Ruidoso, New Mexico. It is a small resort village in Lincoln Forest, a three-hour drive into New Mexico. We will drive, first to Dallas, to dine at the top of the tallest building for our first night. Then we go back to El Paso in time for a night in a hotel, and then on to Ruidoso the next morning. We return to El Paso on a Saturday morning, early enough to settle into our beautiful new one-bedroom apartment at 300 West Schuster Street. It has a pool and is within walking distance from campus. Madly in love, we are finally living our dream.

From the unlikely connection back in 1961 to Susan magically reappearing in El Paso, we are now husband and wife. It is as if our lives are meant to be—*b'shert* in Yiddish.

Our wedding, during which Susan's mom's illness reveals itself through her mere presence, proves to be a metaphor for the rest of our lives. Immense joy and a *simcha*—a celebration in Yiddish—surrounded by a subtext of *tsuris*—Yiddish for trouble or sadness. Even so, Susan, indeed everyone, focuses on the joy of our moment. The love is perhaps expressed in ever more intense joyous energy thrown at us, aware of what lies ahead for her mother.

CHAPTER 4

The Pattern of Our Lives
Up & Down—Life & Death

We focus on the future. I need to get moving. The wedding, my work, and married life have afforded me excuses to avoid some critical stuff. I have not yet applied to law school. Heck, I haven't even taken the LSAT, the law school admission test. In my rush to catch up with life and the arrogance of being an A student, I skip the LSAT prep course. I am not the only one. Many of my friends, also A students, don't bother with the prep class. It should be a breeze for someone like me.

Wrong. I should have studied. My LSAT scores are terrible. Now we wait for the decision from the school, which creates constant tension in our lives. In January of 1967, the letter comes in the mail. "Deferred acceptance." I am on a waiting list! Panic sets in as Susan and I start a what-if game. Before we get too deep into the "what iffing," another letter arrives within a month: "We are pleased to inform you that you have been accepted." Phew.

Back to joy, I'm going to be a lawyer! Thankfully. I believe I will now be deferred from active duty for three years, three years that will be the height of the Vietnam War. I will spend three years in Austin and go into the Army with the rank of captain and an Army lawyer rather than as an infantry second lieutenant, which was my other option.

Susan and I visit Austin during our spring break in March of 1966 to scope it out. Neither one of us had ever been to the campus. Susan's parents want to meet us in Austin, which is a short three-hour drive from Houston.

It is a damp and chilly early March day. The sky is breaking clouds from earlier rains. We drive across the Colorado River to the motel sitting along the water at the opposite river edge. As we walk into a dimly lit lobby, there is a chill in the air. Susan's mom is a specter of her once robust self. She is gaunt. She has trouble walking. Susan stops, and we share a silent gasp as we realize why her dad wanted us to see them. No one knows how long she has. Her breast cancer has spread throughout her body. We share breakfast, though it is hard to look directly at Susan's mom. Despite her diminished physical presence, however, she continues to project both strength and spirit.

Susan's parents spend the next day with us, driving around the campus. They even get out with us and walk around the law school. We take them back to the motel for lunch, send them back to Houston, finish our tour alone, and head back to El Paso.

The pattern of our lives repeats. The ecstatic high of law school admission and my college graduation are replaced with the challenge and tension over our immediate future as Susan's mother gets sicker and sicker. We know now we must be in Houston for the summer to be near Susan's mom. Everyone in the family knows she is not going to survive her breast cancer. Indeed, so does she. The end is inevitable.

No sooner do we have everything set, including an apartment in Houston for the summer, than I get an urgent call to report to the ROTC office. My PMS invites me into his private office and closes the door. "I have some bad news," he tells me. "The Army has denied your request for a deferment to go to law school." He hands me orders to report to Fort Benning, Georgia, for Army officers training right after Labor Day.

He remembers our conversation from two years ago when he said the scholarship would not affect my deferment. He hesitates, eyes the door to be sure it is full closed, pulls out a piece of paper and says: "Sam, I am going to show you something that I am not supposed to because it is classified. You have to promise not to tell anyone." I am confused as I nod my head, yes. I expect the document to be classified by the Army as "SECRET" or something like that. Instead, he shows me a form document pre-printed: "For Official Use Only."

The essential paragraph says that the Army is changing its previous policy and now requires all scholarship recipients to report to active duty. The Army acknowledges that it has changed its mind. It just doesn't want anyone to know.

He then also tells me I can expect orders to head to Vietnam next. He explains that there is a shrinking supply of second lieutenants. I have seen the TV coverage, and it is because they are being killed at a very high rate in Vietnam, sometimes by their soldiers. My PMS wants to help and says he will appeal the decision on my behalf. I don't need to do anything.

My stomach churns before settling into a knot that's pulled tighter and tighter. *What the hell are we going to do?* I wonder. *I barely made it through basic training last summer. I am a heavy smoker, and I am not physically fit. Indeed, I am closer to being a hippy than a soldier.*

What happens if I flunk out of infantry training? Should I desert and leave the country with Susan? I rush home to tell my bride, who is the rock, again. "It will be fine, Sam. You can handle whatever happens."

It doesn't take long for me to hear back that the 4th U.S. Army commander, located in San Antonio, Texas, has denied my appeal. The next step is for my PMS to appeal that decision to the Pentagon.

My panic increases. Law school starts in about one month, and I have orders to report for active duty at Fort Benning, Georgia, in about one month. And Susan's mother just died. I'm skirting a thin edge of emotional collapse, yet I hold it all in as we focus on the loss of Susan's mother.

Sitting now with Susan's family in the Harvest Lane house following her mother's funeral, I again feel alone. We just buried Susan's mother, and I am in a crowd of people I don't know, and I don't know where I will be in only a few weeks from now. I have a sense, too, that within a year, there might be a gathering just like this to mourn me, a casualty of the Vietnam War.

The mourner's meal is the Jewish tradition when a family returns home from a funeral. People I have never met and don't know flow into the house with food and flowers.

"This is Sam, Susan's husband."

"Nice to meet you; sorry it's under these circumstances."

Over, and over, and over again.

I find a seat in the middle of the chaos to isolate myself from the intensity of the room. I prefer the peace of being alone in the middle of the noise, which seems to be more celebration than tragedy.

The telephone rings. A discordant sound. "Sam, it's for you. Your mother is on the phone."

"That's nice," I think. "Mom must be calling to see how I'm doing and to give condolences."

Instead, her voice conveys unexpected urgency. "Sam, I need you to come home! Your father is in the hospital, and he's very sick."

"But Mom, I need to be here with Susan. Her mother just died."

"Sam, *your* family needs you now!"

Her voice has a tone I don't remember ever hearing. For a brief instant, I wonder about the idea of my family versus Susan's family. Even though they are supposed to be one, I know what I must do.

"Okay, Mom. I'll see how fast I can get there. I'll call you once I have the details. I love you."

I hang up, find Susan, and tell her what just happened. Susan's oldest sister, Bernice, is the person most "in charge" at this moment. "We have to get me to El Paso as soon as possible," I tell her.

Flying into El Paso, Texas, over the southwest desert in the summer is an unforgettable experience. The desert heat flows up in waves that buffet the plane. It sways up and down, left and right, and sometimes the plane must circle once or even twice before it lands. The landing is a metaphor for our lives right now.

My oldest sister Marion is at the airport to pick me up when I arrive. She flew in the day before from Washington, DC, where she now lives. Evelyn drove in from Tucson, Arizona, where her husband is now a major in the Army. Harriet and Susie still live at home. We are all here now. We drive to Hotel Dieu Hospital, the same place where I was born. It's smaller than the hospital in Houston, not as modern.

When I walk into my dad's dimly lit room, time slows as everything quiets down within and around me. His bed is to my left, and the room is larger than I expected. The blinds are closed, reminding me of my one visit to Susan's mother in the hospital. Dad is not awake, and I cannot tell if he is just asleep or unconscious. He is lying straight beneath a blue blanket, eyes closed, head up on a pillow. An oxygen mask is over his mouth and nose, and an IV and a heart monitor are attached. A tube comes from underneath the bed to a bag with yellow urine, half-full. He does not move when we enter.

I am, by default, the child-in-charge. Marion and Evelyn, the oldest sisters, need to get back to their homes in other towns. Harriet is in college this summer, and little Susie is just sixteen years old. It seems that I am now "the man in the family."

My schedule is now flexible. My job in Houston is over as I await news from the Army. Will I be deferred to go to law school or head to Fort Benning? In the meantime, I can stay in El Paso and be part of yet another existential vigil with Mom, Susie, and Harriet. Being here in El Paso with the only son's responsibility oddly helps me focus less on my destiny.

Dad regains consciousness periodically. I think he recognizes me, but he isn't oriented, so he just mumbles incoherently. Nurses need to keep him clean, remove the fecal residue, and empty urine bags. They replace IV drips to keep him hydrated. Sometimes when he wakes, he can eat, but someone needs to feed him. Mom doesn't want him to be alone at night, so that becomes my job. We ask for a cot. I will sleep in the room.

I usually arrive for the night at around 8 pm. On the evening of August 13th, Dad seems comfortable when I arrive, just lying peacefully silent in his bed. My routine is to walk up, near his head, touch his forehead lightly, and say, "Hey Dad, it's me, Sam." Some nights I talk to him, though I'm not sure if he really hears me. I recall some of the more memorable times together, especially when I joined him on sales trips in the summers. "Do you remember that lunch in Lordsburg, [New Mexico], when Al [his customer] asked you about the election, and you said, 'Before we talk politics, you should know that I was born a Democrat, and think all Republicans grow horns.' I never forgot that, Dad. I use that line all the time. Perfect for Washington, DC."

Those trips with Dad in the summer taught me many things that I didn't realize until much later in life. In particular, as in that moment in Lordsburg, Al wasn't just a customer. He was Dad's friend. Dad was a successful salesman because his customers became friends—something that, later in life, helped me create a successful business. At this moment, though, I am just trying to make Dad feel better, and in some ways, to build a relationship that never really was. Dad traveled all the time, and he and I never really became close. Indeed, Mom told me how proud Dad is now that I'm about to go to law school. She let me know that while I was in high school, he thought I might end up in jail as a juvenile delinquent.

On the morning of August 14th, Mom and sister Susie relieve me around 9 a.m. I head home to clean up and take care of any business I might have before returning for another night shift. I must look and smell a mess. It takes about half an hour for me to drive back to our home.

The phone is ringing as I walk into the house. I answer to hear my mother's voice. "He's gone, Sam. It happened just after you left. Please get back as soon as you can. Harriet's class will be out on-the-hour, so please pick her up in front of the education building."

I clean up and head over to the University of Texas at El Paso (UTEP) to collect Harriet at the spot she has arranged with my Mom. She is surprised to see me. "What's wrong?" she asks. I tell her that Dad is gone.

As Harriet and I walk down the hallway toward Dad's room, we see Mom and Susie sitting outside in the hallway in chairs next to the door. "The nurses are in the room," Mom tells us. "They're cleaning him up. We can go in when they're finished." As soon as the nurses come out, Mom goes in alone for a few minutes.

"Sam," I hear someone say. I hesitate, perhaps, because of what is about to be my first encounter with a dead body. I hear my name again, maybe from Mom, uttered softly. "Sam, it's your turn." I step slowly into the room, staying as far away from him as I can get, and stare. I'm numb. I don't cry. I feel a mix of anger and regret—a relationship over before it ever began. I replay the angriest moments in my head, along with the things I wanted or hoped for and thought might come with an adult relationship with my father that now won't. His life seems to have been unfair to everyone.

Susan comes in for the funeral. Our El Paso temple is Reform and does not require burial the next day. It takes Susan two days to get here. The funeral is on the third day after death, with a Harding & Orr Funeral Home service and burial in the Temple Mt. Sinai Cemetery. My two oldest sisters arrive. We are all together. I feel the weight of being the one man, with four women, in the family. Mom will be well cared for with her sisters, nieces, and nephews in El Paso.

Susan and I head back to Houston, one week away from our first wedding anniversary and only a few weeks from each of us having lost a parent. I am twenty-two now, Susan is twenty-one. And we do not know where in the world we will be in two weeks since I still don't know if the Army will grant my deferment to go to law school. And in this terrible month, the nation had also suffered one of its first mass shootings on a school campus. On August 1st, a sniper shot and killed nineteen people from the top of the University of Texas tower. We were now worried about our safety in school.

The ordeal takes a toll on me. On Monday, August 22nd, the day before our first anniversary, I'm sick as a dog. Temperature, diarrhea, and nausea. About 3 p.m., I am lying on the couch in the living room taking a nap, not far from the bathroom.

The phone rings. Susan answers, then frantically waves for me to come over to the wall phone. "It's the Department of the Army." I am woozy, in a fog. "Captain Simon," the voice on the phone says. "We are calling to notify you that the Assistant Secretary of the Army has approved your application for a deferment as an exception to standing policy." He hangs up, and I turn to Susan and cry. She hugs me and helps me back to the couch. She never breaks under any pressure. Happy first anniversary. I am going to law school, and I'm not going to die in Vietnam.

Wow. What a summer. What an end to our first year of marriage. In ways we could never imagine, we grew up. Going from two young people—teenagers—getting married and playing house together, we become two young adults facing a complex, exploding world, feeling alone together. The experience of a parent's death, which we've suffered through together, builds a bond between us. Something different and unique.

I sometimes wonder if that could also drive us apart, back to our families. But we don't retreat into our birth families even though that would have been so natural. No, we have already found each other. We are not lost in the world because we have each other. The emotional, existential moments together do not tear us apart. Instead, they knit us together into a form of oneness in a turbulent sea that could easily drown or separate us. We find our joy and security with one another—still newlyweds in some ways—and marching into life together. Oddly, we don't talk about it in these terms. We don't debate it or argue it or feel jealous or second guess. We just do it, are it. We operate as one, working it out, not imagining anything other than us.

CHAPTER 5

Susan's Surgery

The existential roller coaster of 1967, all those years ago—the deaths of two parents, the prospect of becoming cannon fodder of the Vietnam War—wind up being the formative moments of a relationship that we have not understood until now. Susan's uncertain future with Stage 3 cubed breast cancer reawakens Susan and me to the fragility of life.

We call the temple first thing after we arrive home from Dr. Happy's office. After that Friday night Shabbat service, when the rabbi said Susan's name for the first time, we start to let the rest of our family and friends know. Our children are first.

The last either of them heard from us was the "it's just plain old scar tissue" gleeful diagnosis from Dr. Happy. Now we need to tell them that everything has changed—simple and yet complex conversations.

I arrange a lunch with our daughter, who lives in Baltimore, where she is in dental school. She has many medical questions that help me understand what I need to ask about and, to some extent, what to expect. I am surprised at how much general medicine dentists learn. Rachael, I hope, will be able to translate things for us. She is her mother's daughter. She is not panicked or emotional, just matter-of-fact and beautifully wanting to help her dad. She understands that prognoses are hard to make, so she isn't surprised when I say that the doctor's assurances do not convince me that everything will be okay.

Marcus, recently commissioned as second lieutenant in the U.S. Army JAG Corps, is now in Charlottesville, Virginia, at the Army JAG school—the same place I went to thirty years ago and where his sister, Rachael, was conceived. He is in the middle of classes and cannot make it home for a one-on-one conversation, nor can I make the two-and-a-half-hour trip to see him there. Reluctantly, I call him and relay what has happened. I can't tell how he is reacting as the tenor of his voice remains calm.

Next up is the office and my work. I know I will be taking a lot of time off. I need to inform my employees and clients about what is going on. I started Issue Dynamics, Inc., or IDI, in 1986. Over the last fourteen years, the company has grown to nearly fifty people with DC and San Francisco offices.

I speak first with my assistant Eleanor. I know she will steer me through this process and wrap her heart and arms around both Susan and me. With Eleanor's guidance, I find every person—whether staff or client—gracious and committed to helping during this time.

Everything is just about set. One more decision. Should Susan have reconstruction, implants, or just leave her chest flat? Susan and I visit several surgeons and learn that she doesn't have enough extra skin for reconstruction. So, we have no choice—silicone implants it is. Now we wait, and wait, and wait. The surgery is weeks away. I search for ways to express my love to Susan with small gifts presented in unexpected ways. Candy one day, a balloon, a trinket. I love giving her glass and stone hearts from card shops. She gently chides me as she carefully arranges them on the dresser: "Come on, Sam, I will be fine. You don't have to do this."

Our bedtime ritual is for us to set our brand-new Bose clock radio to FM 97.1, a station with a late evening program that allows listeners to call in requests for special occasions or situations. Over several nights, I dial and dial and just get busy signals. A week before the surgery, on the third re-dial, it rings, and the producer answers. I hear the DJ's voice on-air in the background.

I tell the producer about Susan's Stage 3 breast cancer and explain that she will have surgery soon. Our song is "Unchained Melody" by the Righteous Brothers. We fell in love with it the first time we saw the movie *Ghost*. Could they play that song tonight at 11 p.m. and every other night for the next week?

"We can do it tonight, the producer tells me, right after the 11 p.m. news break. You will need to call again, though, to get another dedication. Sorry."

Not a problem. I can make this happen this evening, as a surprise. "Don't fall asleep yet," I say as I keep nudging Susan. "I want you to hear this next song." She is a bit cranky. I just say, "Hush, here it comes. Listen!"

"This next song is for Susan and Sam. They're going through some rough times right now." Then comes, "*Oh, my love, my darling, I hunger for your touch…*"

We hold each other. We enjoy our caresses. I touch Susan's breasts, knowing it will be one of the last times she or I will experience this sensation. We experience deep intimacy. I want to hold her tight enough that we meld into each other. I breathe into her. I inhale her breath into me. Her breath, I realize, is filled with her essence. Not just air nor carbon dioxide, but also the essence of soul interweaving with and into mine. I experience oneness with her. We fall asleep in each other's arms.

The following week, we check into the hospital on a Tuesday at 6 a.m. Susan and I enter the main hospital from the attached garage, with me holding her suitcase, and follow the signs to the operating waiting room. Susan walks to a desk, shows her ID, and has a band put on her wrist with her vital information. They also attach several bright-colored bands indicating her drug and food allergies.

The nurse comes out to usher us into a large area, with busy nurses' stations and dozens of pre-op bays—small areas with curtains around a bed for privacy. Susan's bay is the very first one as we enter. She changes into her hospital gown, and we pack her clothes into the suitcase, which eventually gets tucked under the bed.

I notice, first, that the temperature has dropped. The place is cold. Next, I become aware of how busy and focused everyone is in this area. The staff is readying everything for the operations. Ambient noise from everywhere—families talking, machines whirring, doctors and nurses moving in and out, curtains whooshing open and closed.

It seems like a full house. Each bay has someone in a bed pushed against a wall and shielded with wrap-around curtains. Next to each bed is an IV stand, a heart monitor, and an oxygen mask. One chair for a loved one like me. A nurse call button for patients like Susan.

The nurse comes in to take Susan's blood pressure, pulse, and oxygen level. "It's chilly. Let me get you a blanket," she says. Another nurse pops in, introduces herself, and goes through the chart. "Tell me your name, your date of birth. What procedure will you have today?" She follows the confirmation of Susan's information with, "The doctor will be in to talk with you shortly."

The moment has a strange inevitability about it. We are in a speeding car, and we cannot stop. Thousands of vehicles are all around us. Everything feels urgent and crazy.

I experience an urgent need to do something, to slow time, and think clearly. Instead, I do my best to inject some humor. "Does she have a heart?" I ask the nurse, who is checking Susan's vitals. A polite smile and soft giggle.

The staff acts with great compassion. The nurses, doctors, and aides all notice us and ask about our family. We brag about our kids, the Army lawyer, and soon-to-be pediatric dentist.

Dr. Happy—Dr. John J. Morgan, the breast surgeon—comes into the bay. Still confident, seemingly calm, unhurried, and as always, smiling. His reassuring manner continues as he looks at the chart and the paperwork and asks if we have any questions. We don't. He explains the double mastectomy and the expected three-day hospital stay.

"Please step out for a minute, Sam," Dr. Happy chirps. "I need to mark up the chest area and examine the breasts."

I use the time to wander. I walk by a series of small alcoves arranged in a circle around a central nurse's station. I move slowly around that station and sneak peeks into the other pre-op bays where other families are also getting ready. I make up stories about them. A woman in this next bay, her husband in the chair, and her young son stands next to them: *They must be having something very minor,* I decide. Everyone is smiling. Next bay, all the curtains are closed, yet I still manage to peer inside. An older man seems asleep. An older woman and a younger man are sitting nearby. *It must be his wife and adult son*, I think. *It looks serious.* I walk all the way around and back to Susan's bay, as surgeons and nurses are walking in and out of the various bays I've passed, pleasant and business-like.

It only takes Dr. Happy a few minutes to complete his final review. He pops out of the curtain around Susan's bay. "Everything looks good to go, Sam," he says. "We are starting a sedative right now to calm her down. We will administer the anesthesia in the operating room. The nurses will get you when she is in recovery."

I step back into Susan's little bay with a smile and take Susan's hand. The nurse comes in to tell us they are ready. I stand up, stare down, bend over, close my eyes to kiss her, and once again inhale her breath into me. We say goodbye to her breasts in no particularly ritualistic way. Susan does not even seem sad to see them go.

Two nurses and the doctor open the curtain, step in, and get right to work. One nurse puts up the arms on either side of the bed and unlocks the wheels as the other gets the IV off the permanent stand and connects it to the bed that they are about to move. As they wheel Susan out, the doctor holds the bed railing on the left by her head. I trail behind, reluctant to stop. Susan sees me. I wave as they head down the hall toward swinging doors that lead into the operating room. I stand frozen for a moment, and it seems like forever.

A nurse walks up and touches my arm. "Let me show you to the elevators that will get you up to the main floor and the surgical waiting area."

I had imagined that the surgical waiting area at Inova Fairfax hospital would be private and located near the operating room. Instead, it is on the main floor, right across from the hospital entrance. I step off the elevator and scan the large waiting area for a familiar face. I spot Evelyn, my sister, not far from the entrance doors, off to my right.

I head over, and to my surprise, two rows of seats are filled with family and friends. The rabbi is seated next to Evelyn, who is sitting next to our friends Jan and Soop. They are across from my son and his wife, who sit next to our daughter. Our daughter is next to our cousins, and across from them are more friends. The place seems packed.

They all just smile as if it is perfectly normal, except I didn't know they were coming. I wonder why they are here: For me? For Susan? Perhaps for themselves.

It seems like I should be in charge. I don't know what to do with everyone. We all just sit in silence. No conversation. No mobile phones in 2000. We just sit with an occasional, "Do you want some water? Some coffee?" The clock on the wall captivates me as minutes turn into an hour and then into another hour.

I begin to catastrophize the moment. *Is everything all right?* Susan is allergic to almost every antibiotic on the market. She has many food allergies, including gluten, rice, and seafood. *What if she reacted to the anesthesia?*

I stay seated as my heart rate explodes and my mind races. My feet tap. I replay the conversation with the nurse about the list of allergies. Oddly, I am not too worried about her cancer.

Every time I hear a "ping" telling me that an elevator has arrived on the first floor, I look over, hoping Dr. Happy will walk out. Then it happens. I turn on the ding and see him emerge from the elevators across the room, still in his operating room greens and surgical cap. The mask hangs just under his chin.

I jump up and stride across the room to meet him. We stand off to the side, against the back wall of the waiting room area.

"Susan is in recovery. You can go down now. She is doing as well as can be expected, given the extensive double mastectomy and reconstruction. We sent some tissue to the lab for analysis. The results will be available in about a week."

Everyone is now standing, watching me talk to the doctor. I walk back, share the news, and thank them for coming. Then I head downstairs to recovery.

Susan is in the same bed she was on when they rolled her into surgery. She is semi-conscious, opening and closing her eyes and mainly licking her desiccated lips. Nurses bring a lemon, wet paper towels, and eventually, some orange juice. Susan smiles slightly as if through a haze. She isn't fully awake when the nurses tell me that she is ready to go up to the seventh floor, the cancer floor. I can see her again in the room. Susan and the team squeeze into a nearby elevator marked just for patients. I think it odd that the husband can't be with his wife, the patient.

I walk alone down a long, brightly lit hall, past elevators and hallways, past an overlook above an atrium area on the left and an extensive patient library to the right. I keep moving as the walkway curves around again into a narrow hallway with a new elevator set. These are the elevators to the cancer floor. I press the button for Up. The door opens, so I enter and push the button marked seven. As the elevator begins to move, I realize I don't know Susan's room number.

When I step off the elevator, I enter a new world. The cancer floor has an atmosphere all its own. Slightly confused and uncertain about where to go, I see nothing but a wall in front of me. Room numbers on plaques with arrows pointing in different directions mean nothing since I don't know where to find Susan.

All the rooms on the seventh floor are private. I instinctively turn right and walk slowly past room doors—some closed, others slightly ajar—each with a name on them. I hear a TV as I pass by a small waiting area with what appear to be members of someone's family. I decide the people I see are just waiting their turn, switching with other family members in the room of their loved one right now.

Turning a corner, I almost run into what looks more like a staging area than a nurse's station. I introduce myself to a nurse and ask for Susan Simon's room. She looks at a computer.

"Susan is in Room 735, three rooms down on the right," she says, pointing the way.

I head down the next hallway. The nurses are in the room, helping Susan get comfortable. Every hospital room has a unique aura. Cancer rooms are complicated. There are always a ton of IV stands, monitors, notes, and whiteboards with warnings. I am instantly confused and scared. The back of the bed is up slightly. Susan looks almost white. Small tubes are still poked into her nose; IV lines are connected to her arm. Wires connect Susan to all forms of other machines and monitors. I hear only the rhythm of the ping of the heart monitor.

I can't explain why, or maybe better said, I cannot justify why. I just can't leave Susan alone in this room, as she must now become whole again. Her body, cut and torn, now struggles to heal. I cannot imagine her going through this—the operation and the recovery—by herself. I realize that my job is to be here with her in this room. I stop the nurses as they start to leave. "I am going to stay here with her. Could I get a cot, please?" I am determined that she will not wake up alone, she will not go to sleep alone, and she damned well will not die alone.

I rush home to get a suitcase and throw in some clothes and pajamas. I pack up my computer, work folders, and briefcase. I am in a rush, driven by an urgent desire to get back to Susan. As I speed down the freeway, I make up excuses to use if I get pulled over. Maybe I can convince the cop to escort me to the hospital. "Sir, my wife just got out of surgery, and I need to be with her in case something happens." I don't get stopped.

I put my cot on the right side of the room as I face the bed. It sets close to the ground, about a foot below the top of Susan's bed. In the opposite corner, on the same side of the room, I place a small chair next to a table that can hold my computer. The year is 2000, and nobody has internet access in hospital rooms. I do because one of my clients (Metricom) is deploying one of the world's first wireless internet systems. One of their portable market-trial modems allows me to connect my computer to the internet at 1200 baud. I can be in the room with Susan and keep connected to the office at the same time.

Susan doesn't react well to the anesthesia. She is nauseous all the time. I place one of those small, semi-circle metal containers in front of her when she throws up. I help her get up to go to the bathroom, pushing the IV stand she's tethered to and then help her return to bed.

Two small plastic bulbs hang off each side of her chest in the area near the incision stitches. They fill with a red liquid, drainage from the wound area. The nurses teach me how to empty them. I will need to do this at home by myself since the plastic bulbs will stay in her chest for weeks or maybe even months.

As I do all of this, I smile. My heart melds into Susan ever more deeply. The intimate touch and care of another human have a unique power to animate love. It reminds me of a parent's love for their new and helpless infant. I don't know if Susan has the same experience as I touch her. All I know is that as I engage in caregiving activities, I feel closer to her than I could ever imagine.

I am not nostalgic, pining for better times in the past. It surprises me, though, that I find the physical, spiritual, and emotional courage I need to step up to these new responsibilities. Perhaps all those earlier challenges in our lives have happened to prepare me for this moment.

CHAPTER 6

Growing Up—Living Life

So, in early September 1967, we settle into a duplex in Austin, ready for the start of law school. We are not in Georgia and the Army infantry school.

Susan and I find joy again, despite—or maybe because of—our mutual loss of a parent. We join the Jewish reform temple near campus to fulfill the obligation to recite the mourners' prayer (Kaddish) every Friday night. Meanwhile, we continue our love affair, even as we lead our busy lives. Susan works every day, and I am obsessed with school. I do not take a job during my first year of law school. Instead, I study all the time. I go to class and come home and outline every case in the textbooks—a recommended practice, though no one, except me, ever does it.

My compulsive commitment to study is likely why I do very well in my first year and wind up in the top ten percent of my class. There is a saying about law school: *The first year they scare you to death, the second year they work you to death, and the third year they bore you to death.* All this rings true to both Susan and me as we go through these three years. I manage to stay focused, and by graduation, I qualify for the honor of being a member of the prestigious Texas Law Review. I also graduate with the distinction of membership in "The Order of the Coif," the highest honor for graduating law students at the University of Texas School of Law in 1970.

On our third wedding anniversary on August 23rd, 1969, as that third year of law school begins, Susan and I decide to start a family. We are twenty-four years old and see a bright future—graduate in June and go into the Army as a captain in the Judge Advocate General's Corps. If we time things right, the Army will cover the cost of having the baby. We will soon be reminded of the adage that "people plan, God decides."

In September of 1969, Susan gets off the pill. We think it will take a few months to get pregnant and that the baby likely will be born in August or September after I am on active duty. Well, no, it happens right away, as we discover when she doesn't menstruate in November. I'm ready to spread the news, except Susan won't let me until after the third month. A combination of tradition and caution.

As a fresh decade rolls in, the country itself continues to be in turmoil. My progressive classmates are all vehemently anti-war and anti-establishment. Going right into the Army begins to feel very wrong, yet Susan and I don't see any viable options since she is pregnant with our first child. I do have a close friend who, after getting drafted, deserts to Canada. We can't see ourselves doing that, though we do talk about it.

Then serendipity. A middle ground suddenly appears.

It turns out that one of my law school buddies, Joe-Tom, was a "Nader's Raider," working for Ralph Nader in Washington, DC, this past summer. Joe-Tom approaches me and two of my other classmates, Jim and Peter, then recommends all three of us to Nader.

The opportunity to work with Ralph Nader feels perfect for me. I see this job as what my life should be about, making a real difference in the world. My interview with Nader consists of a thirty-minute phone call to a payphone in Washington, DC, which goes well. I am going to be on the national stage!

It's just like me to be all excited about something that disrupts everything. I call the Army to request a delay in reporting for active duty, and, to my surprise, I get a giant yawn this time. "Oh, you want to wait a bit to come to active duty as a lawyer, Captain? Sure. Take your time." Wow, I didn't expect the request to go so routinely. We need to get going and figure out how we are going to pull this off.

Susan's due date for what we know will be a boy is June 23rd. And I won't be in the Army, which means we have to figure out how to pay for this little guy. But first, I need to get to Washington, DC, study for, and pass the bar exam, which starts June 29th. My start date for my job with Ralph Nader is July 1st. There seems to be no way for me to be present for the birth of our son.

My first child is going to be a boy, a Simon! He will carry the family name forward! Firstborn sons are a big deal in Jewish life. You would think that I would move heaven and earth to make sure that I am with Susan and be among the first to behold, indeed, to hold him. Not me. I am intoxicated with this opportunity to work with Ralph Nader in Washington, DC. I build out a plan-B. Susan's sister Bernice will come to Austin and be with Susan for our first child's birth. I will be in Washington, DC, taking the bar exam.

It turns out that our son is not anxious to enter this world. Like his dad, he will be a bit of a disrupter in life, starting even before being born. June 23rd, the due date, comes and goes with me in DC for the bar exam's final day. I wonder as I take the test if I have become a father. As soon as I finish the last test question, I run to a payphone and call for news. It turns out that our baby is going to need some help. Susan's doctor schedules a Caesarean section for July 1st. Nader is going to have to wait a week. I fly to Austin just in time to be there for the operation.

Marcus. Marcus Bertram Simon. Marcus for my father. Bertram for Bertha, Susan's mother. Marcus, it turns out, is not only his grandfather's name (my dad); we later learn it is also the name of his great-great-grandfather. We, of course, are delighted. The two big "life cycle" events in our short lives have been deaths. Marcus is a celebration. A *simcha*.

We host the bris in the hospital just a few days after he is born, a few days before the traditional seventh day, but I need to get back to Washington. I also need to figure out how to pay the hospital bill. We don't have the $300 in the bank, and they don't take credit cards. After much discussion with the cashier, we are allowed to pay the bill over time.

The birth launches my first year working for Ralph Nader, which proves to be fantastic for Susan and me and baby Marcus, though he doesn't realize it yet. A big moment comes late on a Friday afternoon when Eileen Shanahan of the New York Times is interviewing me about my work. The interview is not going well until Susan, wondering why I am not waiting to be picked up in front of the building, parks and appears at the office door holding baby Marcus. Shanahan looks, melts, and writes a terrific story about my project. She also alerts a feature writer Nan Robertson, about this family with a newborn baby working for Ralph Nader.

A month later, on January 29th, 1971, an article featuring the Simon family—Susan, me, and baby Marcus—appears on the Style Section's front page in the *New York Times*. Titled "Nader Raiding No Plush Job." The article shows Susan holding Marcus up in the air and me at the desk with a pipe in my mouth. It also describes sparse living quarters and our quiet lifestyle. We are celebrities! We all love it.

The calendar, though, dictates our lives. In April of 1971, I need to report for active duty as an Army lawyer. All new Army JAG officers spend several weeks at the Army JAG School in Charlottesville, Virginia, getting oriented to the Uniform Code of Military Justice. The program is attached to the University of Virginia's School of Law.

This new environment provides a welcomed and immediate deceleration of the intense political and policy world of Washington, DC, with Ralph Nader. He's infamous for calling the staff at one or two in the morning. By contrast, in bucolic Charlottesville, we find a basement apartment in a home just outside of the city. We enjoy a lot of idle time together, and our ten-month-old baby Marcus is cute as all get-out. Before we know it, Susan is pregnant again. It looks like the Army will pay for the birth of one of our children after all.

We soon confront another significant life decision. Early in the pregnancy, it appears Susan is going to have twins. The mystery is solved when the x-rays show only one fetus and many rather large fibroid tumors. The doctor raises a related issue. Given the history of cancer in Susan's family, specifically her mother's breast cancer, we should consider removing Susan's uterus.

We didn't plan on a big family. The socially conscious couple that we are, we do not want to contribute to the population explosion. On the other hand, we thought we would have more time to decide—Susan's risk of cancer tips the scale for us. We can always adopt if we want more children.

Rachael Laura Simon is born on November 25th— Thanksgiving day. We name her after Grandma Rosie and my Aunt Lena, the famous lawyer of the family.

Despite a peaceful six-month start that culminates with our daughter's birth, the transition of my work from high-profile Nader advocate to the U.S. Army does not go smoothly, at least for the Army. I write an article critical of the Army's new anti-drug policy published in *The Nation* magazine. The U.S. Army wants to court-martial me for failing to get my article approved in advance. Thanks to the Judge Advocate General's intervention on my behalf, the official punishment is only a letter of reprimand in my personnel file and an off-the-record "attaboy" from the JAG himself.

Soon after this incident, I am offered a transfer to the U.S. Army's Office of Chief Trial Attorney in Washington, DC, where I will be able to direct my energy toward suing cheating government contractors. It is the best job in Army JAG and a chance to get back to Washington, DC.

The rhythm of our lives, Susan and me. Soar and slide. Up and down. Fall in love and lose our parents. Have two children and worry about uterine cancer. I almost get court-martialed and then transfer to the best job in Army JAG.

CHAPTER 7

Existential Experiences

*W*e reinstall ourselves in a Northern Virginia suburb of Washington, DC, following eighteen eventful months at Fort Lee, Virginia. Life feels routine for our family of four when, in the Spring of 1973, I receive a call from my Aunt Etta, my mother's oldest and only remaining sister. The tenor of her voice tells me there's a problem.

"Sam, you need to come home. Something is wrong with your mother."

Aunt Etta explains that Mom is hospitalized and is having trouble with her mind. The doctors suspect dementia but are not sure. The Army grants me emergency leave, and I head to El Paso. I call my sisters and promise to let them know what I find as soon as I get there.

Mom is in a private room in Hotel Dieu Hospital. The same hospital where my dad died seven years ago. I am nervous and shaken when I visit her. She is semi-conscious, disheveled, and not fully covered. I see things a son shouldn't.

She begins to talk, seemingly reliving her past: "Come inside, Rose, it's time to come inside." Rose is one of her sisters who died some forty years ago.

The neurologist drills a hole into Mom's head to remove fluid that has accumulated there. "Yes, it's dementia," he declares after the hospital runs a test on the liquid. I'm skeptical. Everything about the neurologist feels condescending, as if she is trying to prove to me, an interloper, that she was correct from the beginning.

I fill in my sisters and share my reservations about the quality of my mother's medical care. None of us is comfortable with what has happened in El Paso. We all agree we need a second opinion, so we arrange to have Mom seen at the Mayo Clinic in Rochester, Minnesota, where they have a new, state-of-the-art machine called an MRI. It doesn't take long to get the news—Mom's breast cancer has reappeared in her brain.

How can that be? Even with the death of Susan's mom, my mother's breast cancer event was not a defining moment in my life. Everyone said it was minor in one breast and that the mastectomy was "precautionary." The operation happened over the first summer I spent in Houston. Two years ago, my mom hit that so-called "magic five-year" point and was declared "breast cancer-free." Now, breast cancer is in her brain.

I now believe—no. I now *know* that breast cancer always kills. In my view, breast cancer, despite the broad claims of great modern treatments, has no cure. This claim that after five years, cancer is gone, is fiction. Now the doctors explain that the breast cancer indeed has spread into Mom's bloodstream. Now we just wait. The verdict is clear; her condition is terminal—no further treatment is possible.

We move Mom directly from Mayo to live with my sister Evelyn in McLean, around the corner from where Susan and I now live. We all want to make the most of the time that Mom has left.

On September 5th, 1973, we check Mom into a semi-private room at the George Washington Memorial Hospital in the District of Columbia. We know we are getting toward the end, and the doctors ask us what level of care we want for her at the end. Medical directives have not yet become commonplace, so we, the five children, need to decide what to do when she begins to stop breathing. Evelyn and I agree not to take extraordinary measures and confirm that decision with our sisters Marion, Harriet, and Susie.

Midafternoon on September 8th, we get a call from the hospital telling us that the end is near. A flashback for me to Houston and Susan's mom six years ago. I immediately head down to George Washington Hospital, a fifteen-minute drive from our home, just inside the District of Columbia off the Roosevelt Bridge. My sister Evelyn will join me as soon as she can get away from home. Last time, when it was Susan's mom, I wasn't welcomed in the room; now, it might be just me.

The semi-private room is empty as I enter slowly, trying not to make noise. Mom's roommate has disappeared, the other bed in the room is empty. I am alone with my mother. The room is silent. The only noise I hear comes from down the dim hallway. I see, more than hear, the short quick breaths coming from Mom. It is getting late, and the sun is going down. Her breathing turns softer and less frequent. Anxious, I grab the phone in the room to call my sister, Evelyn. I hear the frustration in her voice as I urge her to hurry. Something is going on at home, and she is having trouble getting out the door. "I'm leaving now, Sam. I'll be there soon, depending on the traffic. I am so sorry."

As I hang up, two nurses walk into the room, and I introduce myself as the son. They greet me without stopping. One moves to the right side of the bed, the other to the left. I move to stand at the foot of the bed, not knowing what to expect. I want to find internal strength. After all, I am now the man in the family. I do not feel so strong right now. I have never been in the presence of a human being as they take their last breath, and here I am now with my mother, alone.

I don't hear an orchestra playing. There is just silence. I watch the two nurses face each other on opposite sides of the bed. They each gently take hold of a wrist to feel for a pulse. There is no heart monitor, and there are no sounds, just two nurses holding a wrist, seemingly counting down. Almost as if the nurses have choreographed the moment, they simultaneously look up, nod, put the wrist down, and turn to me. "She's gone," one of them says.

I feel unmoored and gasp for air. An irrepressible urge to demand that the nurses do something wells up in my chest. My being does not want this moment to be. DO SOMETHING. DO SOMETHING! HELP HER BREATHE. DON'T LET HER DIE! A primordial scream builds in my chest, yet sticks in my throat.

My eyes begin to fill with tears. I slowly start to turn away when out of the corner of my left eye, I notice a giant swirl, a spinning tuft of a cloud. The cloud has thin strands of transparent whiteness—billions of them—in different shapes and lengths. Spinning. Spinning.

The swirl is perhaps five feet from bottom to top and inches or maybe only millimeters thick. The center material comes together in a puffy pointed end and then strings back into the gossamer circle. The material is thinnest in the center of the swirl and denser at the outer edges, yet the tuft strands remain transparent.

I feel the temperature in the room drop. As I move slowly—almost floating—I turn toward my left. The material, which behaves as if it has an intention, swirls in perfect form from right to left. It stutters for an instant as if noticing me, then streaks out of the room so fast there should be a "whoosh." Instead, there is only silence.

My head jerks around as my mother's soul exits this dimension of time and reality. The journey is over. Mom is gone.

I can't breathe, and yet I am full of breath. My eyes explode with tears. The nurses, still standing facing each other, notice me. One quickly walks up and takes me by the arm to guide me from the room.

The moment scares and confuses me. I know I am not supposed to see what I just saw.

It is my first experience with the supernatural. I know what people call people who hear and see things in their heads that nobody else can hear or see. Is that what happened here? *Have I hallucinated?* I wonder. *Is this just my grief talking?*

I have since come to believe that my experience with my mother, as her life force exits at her last breath, is a blessing. This gift was her way of saying goodbye to me. At the time, though, I am scared and confused.

I do not tell anyone about the experience, not Evelyn, not the nurses, not even Susan. The fear and confusion do not leave me. Instead, the experience creates a sense of guilt and of humility that preoccupies my mind for years.

CHAPTER 8

Preludes

*I*n the year 2000, I am sitting with Susan in her hospital room after her double mastectomy. Yes, it was many years ago that I was in my mother's room, and yes, that experience still sits in my heart. Indeed, that instance of revelation teeters even today on the edge of my awareness.

Now I help Susan vomit, go to the bathroom, and drain the fluids from the plastic bulbs filling with red liquid on each side of her chest. Maybe I am just tired tonight, or perhaps I've been in this room too long, whatever the reason I become overwhelmed. The sense of intimacy disappears as my certainty of her end erupts. My head bursts as my heart screams, *I cannot do this! I don't want to do this! I do not do this stuff well!* Hell, I hardly ever changed our kids' diapers, and now I am helping Susan vomit. I really, really don't want to be here.

I look at the door, look at the cot, look at that semicircular metal pan just waiting for her to get sick again. Then in an infinite moment, time stops. I exit the present, transported to a different yet parallel dimension and time. No one else notices. The physical reality of my presence at that moment does not change. I am at once here in Susan's hospital room and yet somewhere else.

I am in the center of an empty grand ballroom, unsure exactly where I am in relation to everything around me. I see, or perhaps become aware of, a high ceiling with blinding spotlights, empty chairs around small tables that fill the space on all sides of the dance floor, even in front of a platform on one side that is large enough for a good-sized orchestra of forty or fifty or maybe even more musicians. The very back of the ballroom lies in semidarkness, with doorways opening into a brilliant white glare that never makes it into the ballroom itself. It is as if a permeable white sheet hangs over the exit.

What's happening to me? I wonder. At first, I think it is a nightmare. Yet, I am not asleep. I shake my head, pinch my arms. Maybe a daydream?

As stark and abrupt as this moment is, I am not afraid. Tangible calm envelopes me. A sense of the sacred, of the profound, of deep internal peace. I am where I am supposed to be at this moment. As I wander around this brilliant ballroom, I am filled with awe. The ballroom sits empty, hollow, pregnant with purpose and readiness. I am the only one here.

The moment ends as abruptly as it started, and I am back in room 735, on the seventh floor of Inova Fairfax

Hospital. In that moment of return, my soul is enveloped by the inevitable certainty that this ballroom has a particular purpose and that I alone know that purpose. This ballroom is waiting, waiting for Susan—for Susan and me to walk out onto the dance floor, to embrace and begin the final ritual dance, swaying through time until she simply evaporates into a wisp of white swirl exiting through the bright lights into eternity.

The experience is new, yet I've always sensed that this place, this ballroom, or something like it, exists. It evokes a deep feeling of knowing that every other existential experience of my life happened in order to prepare me for this coming moment. It answers the question I do not want to answer, that I am afraid to have answered for me. The unthinkable that I now must think. The unimaginable that I must now imagine. How to hold the one I love most in the world, my "meant to be," the love of my life. How do I comfort and embrace her as she takes her last breath and slips into eternity?

It will be in this place—the ballroom. I believe in this place, this ballroom space. I have been here before—though I didn't realize it—in 1973, during that infinite moment as my mother said goodbye on her way to eternity. I understand that the tuft, that momentary stutter so many years ago, was real and a prelude to now.

CHAPTER 9

Good News

*T*hree days later, and notwithstanding my moment of terror in the ballroom, Susan has slowly and steadily regained her strength and stability. The nurses now encourage her to walk around the long oval hallway that winds around the seventh floor. I enjoy walking with her.

It takes a bit to get ready. The IV stand needs to be unlocked so it can roll down the hallway. Susan works hard to get her robe on. She fumbles around before she can slide her right arm through one sleeve. I try to help and get swatted away, though she needs me to wrap the other sleeve around her shoulder over the IV line. We move to the doorway of her room and pause before we walk into the hallway. We look both ways to avoid colliding with other patients also walking the hall to get stronger.

The hallway divides naturally as if a two-way street with traffic moving in opposite directions. We walk forward on the right; people heading toward us are on the left. Over time, we begin to recognize each other, smiling and nodding as we pass in the hall. We usually check in with the folks we see. "Is the arm feeling better?" "When are you going home?" "Oh, sorry to hear that. Hope I can avoid that complication." I call it 'hallway chitchat.'

Over time we begin to feel part of a club, 'The Seventh-Floor Club.' Still, I sometimes secretly root for Susan to speed-walk past the others. I want her to be here to win this race that my heart has already told me she can't.

Today, the third day since the mastectomy, Dr. Happy appears at Susan's door at 7 a.m., before Susan and I have had a chance to take our walk. Indeed, I am still in my PJs.

"Good news!" he almost shouts. His demeanor is living up to his nickname. "Got it all, Susan! Got it all, Sam! First, we found very little additional cancer in the right breast, and in the left breast, we found nothing!"

He takes a breath. I look at his face and wonder if he is about to explode. "And the *best* news of all." He pauses and then nearly screams out, "The truly *best* news is that the lab found no cancer in Susan's lymph nodes." Dr. Happy is almost ecstatic.

Suddenly, I become acutely aware that I have been grossly negligent in this breast cancer journey, unlike the last cancer scare when I called Ralph Nader and Dr. Sid Wolf. This time, I have done nothing but ask friends for their recommendations for cancer doctors. The internet is still nascent. Google is new. I do not buy books to become an expert on breast cancer. Susan learns most of what she knows from her friends who have breast cancer or are acquainted with people who have had it. We don't even know enough to have asked the right questions. It is as if I know it doesn't matter because the end is predetermined.

Dr. Happy explains that for breast cancer to metastasize from Susan's breast to other organs in the body, it needs to travel through a series of lymph nodes, specifically those located under the arm and along the side of the breast area. If the lab finds no cancer in the lymph nodes, then the probability is high that the cancer is confined to the breast area. If they find cancer in the lymph nodes, though, then the probability is high that cancer has transited throughout the rest of the body.

For me, hearing that no cancer is in Susan's lymph nodes turns everything I have come to "know" on its head. What I "know" in my heart is not written in books. Susan's mother died from breast cancer, and my mother died from breast cancer. Susan is going to die from breast cancer. I do know that.

Today though, I let my guard down. *Maybe this isn't a death sentence after all.*

Susan continues to gain strength and wants me out of her room. I'm often in the bathroom at night when she wants to get in, and then we bump into each other. She is also worried about me and can tell I'm anxious. "Sam, you need some real rest, and you need to get back to the office! Go home, sleep, then go to work. I will be fine." Dr. Happy eyes me in my pajamas and messed up hair and agrees with Susan. I think everyone, including the nurses, agrees with Susan and will be glad to see me go.

I reluctantly pack up and head to our house. I feel guilty. Once there, I spend my time getting ready to bring Susan home. My style, not hers, is *what if*.

What if she can't make it up the fourteen stairs to the master bedroom? How will she get onto our king-sized bed? The bed is so high off the floor that she already struggles to get her butt onto the top of the mattress. What if she can't do that now?

What foods do I need to have in the house? Who will cook? Do I need a home nurse?

I also must focus on medicine and wound care. I still need to empty the two plastic bulbs attached to each side of Susan's chest, right above the incision of where the breasts used to be, as they fill with pinkish liquid. I will need a system to make sure she takes her pills on time. Of course, I have to ensure that I'm available for follow-up doctor's appointments.

Exactly one week after her surgery, Susan is ready to come home. I am in awe of her strength and determination, which shows up immediately upon her arrival when she sets a rule for friends who want to visit. They are not allowed in the house unless they can be one-hundred-percent positive. No tears, no fears. *Celebrate the new Susan* is the rule of the house. It applies to me too. No matter how I feel—how sure I am that something terrible is about to happen—I stay positive in Susan's presence.

A few days later, a lab report arrives in the mail. Not expecting it, I tear open the envelope before Susan knows it has come. Remember, Susan wants to hear good news only.

Yes, more good news! I stare at the black and white bold print at the top of the report: *No cancer evident in the lymph nodes.* It is as if the lab knows this is good news and wants to make sure I see it first.

Hospitals, of course, can't say anything in just seven words. I stare at a page and a half of fine print. My eyes skim over it. Blah blah blah, *The conclusions are subject to the results of chemical and dye tests, which will be available in approximately one week.* None of that tiny print registers. My eyes glaze over the words. I experience the report as unexpected good news.

I run upstairs, show the report to Susan, and reread the sentence, "no cancer evident in the lymph nodes."

"See, Sam, I told you so! Everything is going to be just fine!"

My nagging reluctance to accept any good news is being tested. I even run into Dr. Happy the next day in the parking lot of our local grocery store. It turns out he lives nearby, and he shops there from time to time. He sees me from two parking aisles over and shouts out my name. "Hey, Sam!" About three other people named Sam turn toward the voice, including me. I am surprised to see him. He waves and then spreads out his arms wide and gives a big two-thumbs-up with a great big Dr. Happy smile.

Two-thumbs-up. Maybe, just maybe, I am wrong about how this 'story' will end. Maybe everything will be okay. We can live just fine with the implants.

Everything is looking up in the week since Susan's return from the hospital. At home, she just gets stronger. She climbs the fourteen stairs from the main floor to our master bedroom relatively easily. The only indication that she just had major surgery is that she enjoys a midafternoon nap.

Even I'm doing a little better. I empty the liquid-filled plastic bulbs without hesitation. As time passes, less and less liquid flows, with the bulbs collecting just a trace at the end of most days—a sign that Susan is healing.

CHAPTER 10

Everything Changes

*I*n the ten days that follow Susan's double mastectomy, a new routine enters our lives. Susan's strength and stability are remarkable. Today is the date for her first post-surgery appointment, set as part of the hospital's check-out routine. The bandages need to be changed, the incisions checked, and a few minutes with Dr. Happy. We hop into the car for the now familiar drive to Doctor Happy's office and arrive, walking with positive energy in our steps.

We know more treatment lies ahead. Today, we expect Doctor Happy to clear Susan to see an oncologist, who will decide if Susan will need chemotherapy or radiation treatment. With this last report and Dr. Happy's parking lot thumbs-up, we hope further treatment may not be necessary or at least just precautionary. With no cancer in the lymph nodes, this might just be all the treatment Susan needs. The boobs are gone, and the cancer is gone, or so we expect.

Dr. Happy's office is now familiar, and the staff recognizes us as we enter. A nurse comes to take Susan back to the exam room to remove the plastic bulbs. No more fluid in the last twenty-four hours. Dr. Happy does not even need to examine her. Instead, the nurse comes out to get me while Susan is getting dressed. She joins me as we walk back to Doctor Happy's private office.

As we walk into the room, it is apparent that Dr. Happy is not happy. At first, he is silent, a reaction opposite to his demeanor when he bounded into Susan's hospital room that early morning to give us the "good news." My emotional radar lights up, and I return to the moments in the narrow, closet-like room when he told us Susan's cancer was Stage 3.

He seems reluctant to start. "Um. Well. Uh." Then, "The chemical and dye reports are in and, uh, uh, and I am afraid that the lab did find extensive cancer in Susan's lymph nodes. They tested seventeen nodes, and cancer is in ten of them."

A brief pause for us to absorb the news. Then, before we react, Dr. Happy starts again with another series of sounds. "Humm, err, uhh …. Well, the lab said they made a mistake in the first place. I had them go back and look at the slides, and they told me that the cancer was evident in the slides they had looked at during the surgery. They just missed it." Dr. Happy's reassuring presence has transformed into a reluctant, apologetic presenter of bad news.

Once again, he doesn't pause for a response, nor does he ask if we have any questions. Instead, he fills what has become an uncomfortable, albeit brief, silence with, "Have you picked an oncologist?"

We tell him we are in the process and mention that Doctor Alan Blonder comes highly recommended by several of our friends. Dr. Happy knows him well and confirms that he is one of the most respected members of the largest oncology practice in the Northern Virginia area. The oncology practice is associated with Inova Fairfax Hospital, where Susan had her mastectomy. "Dr. Blonder would be an excellent choice," he concludes.

Susan and I drive home in silence. The weight of the moment is too great to allow either of us to speak, though I suspect I am projecting my burden onto Susan. She has to know, as do I, that the future has changed dramatically.

Once home, we walk silently into our dining room, pull out two adjacent chairs, turn them to face each other, and sit in silence. No words, just looking at each other in the dim light of late day. We could have turned on a light. It just doesn't seem right. *We need to decide what to do with the rest of our lives,* I think. This news reaffirms for me what I have come to know. This story of Susan's cancer is not going to end well.

My voice breaks the silence of the moment. "Susan, we need to decide how we want to live the rest of our lives together." I wait for a response, which doesn't come. She just looks lovingly into my face. "Let's put everything on hold for a bit, and travel, see the world, go to all those places we always talk about."

Susan takes her time, along with a deep breath, then scoots her chair closer to me and looks me in the eye. "Sam, I have only one thing I need to do right now, and that is to beat this thing." Another pause and, "If we do not love the life we love right now, then let's change it. Not because I might die, but because we don't want to live this life. Are you unhappy with our lives?"

Her question flusters me. Before I figure out how to reply, she continues. "I'm not. I love this life, and I want to keep living it with you."

I love this woman. I know she will not "beat this thing." This steely determination is, in part, why I love her so deeply. I don't want her to be wrong; I wish I were wrong. Yet, I know that I am not. I take her hand. We stand up, hold each other for a minute, and return to our evening routine.

Three days later, a new report comes in the mail. I open it and flip through the details of what we already know, now described in a written laboratory report: *seventeen nodes tested, ten with cancer*. On the last page, though, are words, words that I will never forget. *On further review, the diagnosis is changed.*

Well, the diagnosis may have changed for the lab, but it is not for me. I never really believed that first report. Yes, I allowed myself a momentary slip, permitting myself to think maybe this wasn't a death sentence after all. For just an instant, I fell for my façade. The same face I know I must keep until the end. I kick myself for even

pretending to myself for just an instant that everything—
or anything—would work out.

There is more news about the chemistry of Susan's breast
cancer. I learn that chemical markers inside cancerous
breast tissue indicate the likelihood of recurrence and
spread. Of course, with cancer in Susan's lymph nodes, we
know that it has traveled through the nodes into the rest
of her body.

The chemical markers are indicators of whether Susan's
breast cancer's spread can be slowed by medicine. If the
breast tissue with cancer tests positive, then the breast
cancer spread can be suppressed by drugs like Tamoxifen.
If the breast cancer tissue tests negative, there are no drugs
to reduce the likelihood of recurrence or spread. The report
makes clear that all of Susan's markers are "negative"—
Tamoxifen is useless.

I don't run to show this report to Susan. Instead, I
once again exit reality. In a blink of the eye, I am in the
ballroom, the inexplicable split-screen—myself standing
in the den, holding the piece of paper, staring at this
updated report while I suddenly awaken in this other
place in time and space, the ballroom.

*Everything is clear now as I stand in the center of the
dance floor of that grand, elegant ballroom. The air is thin.
I can barely breathe. Everything is indistinct except for the
brilliant lights over the dance floor. Time is frozen as all the
musicians who will play the music for our dance now enter
the ballroom. Violinists, cellists, two bass players, clarinetists,*

flute and piccolo players, even a harpist with a giant instrument appear. On and on and on, walking past me as if I don't even exist. The musicians each know their task. They each know the song they will play for our dance even though Susan isn't here. Yet.

It is time now for us to pick the oncologist. Susan doesn't think this is an issue, "Sam, let's just go with Doctor Blonder. Jim recommends him, and so does Dr. Happy." Jim is a family friend and an executive at Inova Hospital System in charge of community relations.

My instinct is different. I want to find the best breast oncologist in the world for Susan, perhaps the only way to "beat this thing." My determination to get Susan to the best cancer center in the world grows after I speak with my internist. Susan and I have had different internists since we have been married. It was usual as we grew up for a man and a woman to have separate doctors. As it happens, I have an annual physical appointment scheduled shortly after this last visit with Doctor Happy. I want to make sure I stay healthy.

As my doctor goes through his routines, I fill him in on Susan's breast cancer and the news that it is in her lymph nodes. I have been seeing him for twenty years, and he knows me well. He gets right to the point. "It doesn't matter, Sam. What they don't tell you," he says in his unique doctor's voice, "is that the cancer cells are sub-microscopic, thus so small that they will have already spread throughout the body by the time they are detectable by current technology." In other words, he says, cancer is everywhere inside Susan and probably has been for some time. It just isn't awake everywhere. Yet. "What we don't know is what triggers the cancer cells to wake up and start growing again." He means to comfort me, but I am not encouraged.

Once I get home, I confront Susan with my firm conviction that we should consider a world-class cancer center for her treatment. Why not Mayo, or Memorial Sloan Kettering, or MD Anderson in Houston, her hometown?

No, Susan is adamant. She doesn't want to be away from home, and, yes, we argue. I remind her that after her previous biopsy, Inova Fairfax Hospital had to send her breast tissue to Mayo Clinic. Why not just go to Mayo? She is adamant. I compromise. We can go with Dr. Blonder if we get a second opinion here in the DC area. We need to talk to at least one other doctor, just to be sure.

One of Susan's friends from our temple, Joan, who also has breast cancer, including in her nodes, recommends an oncologist in Washington, DC. She and her husband, Stan, swear by the doctor. Susan and I agree to check out both Doctor Blonder and Joan's oncologist.

I've never thought much about the process of selecting a doctor, much less an oncologist, until now. Yet, when the issue is life or death, it becomes *the* question. How the hell do you pick a *cancer doctor*? A doctor whose judgment, skill, and training may determine whether you—or the person you love—will live or die? Even with our two appointments scheduled, I continue to reach out to friends for advice. I soon learn that many of our friends have or had cancer, and, like Joan, they all swear by their doctor. And no two people seem to have used the same one.

Even with these recommendations, I still want to take Susan to the Mayo Clinic, Memorial Sloan Kettering in New York, or MD Anderson in Houston. Or somewhere, anywhere else. I think maybe, just maybe, if we go somewhere else, things will turn out differently.

Susan won't have any of this running all over the country. I think I can be more persuasive once she meets these local doctors. I'll hold my fire for a bit. We get an evaluation appointment with the oncologist recommended by Susan's friend, Joan, within the week. His office is in Washington, DC, near where I work, not near where we live. His affiliation is with George Washington Hospital, the same hospital where my mother died.

We also schedule an appointment with Dr. Blonder for a few days later. Dr. Blonder seems a more logical choice. His practice is in Virginia and closer to our home than Joan's doctor, and Dr. Blonder's practice is affiliated with Inova Fairfax Hospital. Dr. Happy recommends him. Perhaps because I sense Susan will like him, or maybe because I'm exhausted, our interview with him does not go very well. I challenge him from the start. "If we don't do something different and out of the box, I know how this story is going to end. Don't you?" I can hear my voice getting louder, almost a scream.

I begin to cry, and as Susan comforts me, I try to talk but can't get the words out. It begins to sink in—despite my desperate urge to find someone, anyone, who will fix everything now—that I do not get to decide. My job is *not* to be the director.

My job? My job is to be the supporter. I am the other half of that which makes us—Susan and me—complete. And when else in our lives is it more vital for us to be whole than when *our* body is badly broken?

At this moment, sitting in Dr. Blonder's office, next to Susan, me crying, I come to understand how deeply intertwined I am with Susan, just how much I love her, and that I am about to lose her. No matter what has happened before, no matter what I have ever said or thought about us, now, at this moment, I understand our singularity, our knitted-together essence of a unique being. God breathed life into Adam and Eve, and that enabled God to speak them into being. We have spoken us—Susan and me—into being, each the equal half of the other, through our life together.

Now, I am in mortal fear of being torn apart. I cannot stand the thought, nor imagine the pain.

We arrive for Susan's first examination with Dr. Blonder shortly after we make our decision. We enter his office and immediately run into Gregg and Tybee, friends from the temple, as they are leaving. It confuses me. I recognize Gregg. I wonder who the woman is with him. Then I realize it is his wife, Tybee. We didn't know that Tybee was sick. She looks just awful. Gaunt, hollow cheeks, eyes sad, and hair that had always looked neatly coiffed now just hanging straight down to her shoulders. No wonder I didn't recognize her.

How did we not know? I look at Susan, who, with her eyes, replies with the same question. Tybee, we learn, has metastasized ovarian cancer.

The moment with Tybee and Gregg reinforces the ambiance and aura of the dark, unhappy waiting room.

We sit in silence until a nurse comes out and calls Susan's name. It takes Susan a moment to respond, and she stands slowly. I notice her hesitancy in a nanosecond. I immediately pop up, startling Susan, and whisper to her, "I am coming with you! You are not doing this alone." The nurse doesn't seem to notice our little interchange. Susan doesn't have time to object, even if she wanted to.

We follow the nurse out of the waiting area down the hall into a narrow, long treatment room. Susan and I enter the room with caution. It's cold for me. Susan seems fine with the temperature. She walks toward the exam table and sits down. I stand next to her. Dr. Blonder raps his knuckles on the door, turns the handle, and walks right in with a "hello."

He tells Susan to take off her blouse and a halter top that covers her bandages. The doctor then gently unwraps the dressing, slaps the top of the exam table, inviting Susan to lie down. Her chest is bare, revealing the incision's dark lines still held together with slightly swollen, purplish, and puffy stitches at the center.

I stare uncomfortably, not knowing if I should avert my eyes—except I can't. How strange to watch as another man puts his hands on Susan's bare chest. Susan doesn't seem to mind. I marvel at her ability to let Dr. Blonder touch her so intimately and not react. I wonder if she would have preferred a woman doctor. I never asked. I don't yet realize that Susan has no sensation at all in what was the breast area of her chest. It will take me a while to remember not to fondle the implants.

As Dr. Blonder lets his fingers slide along the lips of the incisions, he suddenly stops. His finger freezes in place at one specific spot on the incision line. He stands up straight without saying a thing, does a military-style about-face, and marches over to a telephone on the wall at the far end of the room near the door. He picks up the phone and starts to talk.

Wow, that's weird, I think. I move closer to Susan, standing in the space that Dr. Blonder has just vacated. Susan and I look at each other, then at him, then back. *Did he hear his name paged in the muffled sounds of the office loud-speaker system?* I wonder. I close my eyes and strain to listen to the sounds echoing in the hall just outside the room. *Maybe he recognized his name.* On the phone, he speaks to someone in a low voice. Oddly, even in this small exam room, I cannot make out a word he says. I look at Susan, who merely shrugs her shoulders.

He hangs up the phone, spins around, and strides toward us with great purpose. He puts his finger back down on Susan's chest and presses it against the scar tissue as if massaging something. He stops and looks up. He is just confirming what he had felt before. "I have found a lump on Susan's chest here at the incision point, and it needs to be looked at right away," he says. "I have made an appointment for Susan with Dr. Morgan, the breast surgeon, for tomorrow at 9 a.m. You need to see him."

That is what he was doing on that phone, making the appointment. And he is not happy.

We leave without saying much. Susan is once again stoic. "Everything will be okay, Sam. Don't worry."

I don't respond. I know the end of this story already. I always have.

The route to Dr. Happy's office is familiar; this trip, though, is not routine. When we walk into an exam room, he puts up an x-ray of the area and looks at what even I now recognize as a lump. He has Susan lie down and opens her blouse. Another man's hands on her chest. His face tells it all.

He asks a nurse to call and find out how soon he can get an operating room. It doesn't matter where the facility is located, provided it is within the Inova system. It turns out that Inova Fairfax Hospital, the one near our home and where Susan had her mastectomy and stayed for that first week, does not have an operating room available for the next ten days. He doesn't want to wait that long. He can get into Inova Fair Oaks, a sizable outpatient facility about fifteen miles further away from our home. Dr. Happy books the procedure for the following Friday.

Dr. Happy is also clearly not happy. And I am not happy.

CHAPTER 11

Getting Ready—Seeking Help

*B*ack at home, a strange silence settles in between us about what just happened, permeating the space of our lives. Susan doesn't alter her routine. I cannot speak of the gigantic hole that has opened in the center of my being. Despite how certain I have felt that Susan will suffer the same fate as her mother, the moment has never felt so imminent. Perhaps up to now, it was just a theory in my mind, self-indulgence on my part. Thinking she will die allows me to feel sorry for myself. Oh, poor me. No, I do not believe I am that self-absorbed, yet Susan's end has become dramatically more real. It is within sight. I think about it every time I look at Susan.

I tend now to get up early most Sunday mornings. Careful not to wake Susan, I tiptoe downstairs and walk around our McLean, Virginia, home. These early Sunday mornings are also the times I tend to get sad and depressed. I can because Susan doesn't see me. She is still in bed, upstairs.

As I wander through the predawn, silent house, I wonder what life will be like being alone. I have never lived alone. I grew up in a house filled with people. Even with Dad constantly on the road, we always had people around. Four sisters, Mom and Dad, equaled seven people in a house with three bedrooms. Then add my Grandmother Alfman for a few years and my Aunt Julia for many years. Lots of people around all the time. I lived at home in that house with my family until I got married and moved out to live with Susan.

As I walk around these Sunday mornings, I sense a great emptiness that lurks around the corners of the predawn darkness. This fear is not just about living alone; the fear is about *being alone*. The anticipation of losing part of myself will create an existential aloneness in the universe. Like floating through space between stars and planets without oxygen. A place of ballrooms and orchestras. Angels and souls. A place of being alone.

As I walk around the house this early Sunday morning, I stop at my laptop computer that sits atop a high countertop between our kitchen and den. The laptop suddenly wakes up as if it sees me. A bright screen with AOL's Instant Messenger presents itself. I bend down to see the screen and notice Susan's sister-in-law Roz's username BubbieRoz. She's online. I bend down and type, "You there?"

She responds, "Yes. How is Susan doing?"

I try to tell her that Susan is not doing very well.

"Don't worry," she tells me. "Everything is going to be just fine!"

Of course, Bubbie Roz is going to say that. She had breast cancer three years ago, and she is doing just fine. If she were in the room, I would have yelled: "Don't you know not everyone does *just fine!*"

I tell her about the post-mastectomy lump and the procedure to remove it that we scheduled for this Friday.

"Should Melvin come up?" she asks. Melvin and Roz are the members of her family closest in age to us.

I type back, "I think he will want to be with his baby sister." Roz seems to understand the import of these words.

Roz is the first person I've told about the lump. I slowly close the laptop, folding the screen down tight. As I straighten up, tears fill my eyes, and again, time stops.

I have returned to the ballroom, except now I am standing in the center of the dance floor. The remaining members of the orchestra have made their way onto the orchestral riser. The instruments are coming out of their cases now. The noise of all the different musical instruments being warmed up simultaneously and in different ways is deafening and cacophonous.

I don't understand what is going on with me. Visions? Dreams? Sounds. Images. Out-of-body experiences? I shudder as a deep fear grips my gut. Nausea sweeps over me.

I realize that I need help. Doctor's appointments, stiff-upper-lip, working again every day and pretending that nothing bad is about to happen to Susan.

Standing in our beautiful home, alone, the future clear in my mind, I realize that I cannot possibly do what I now know I will have to do.

I need help. I need to talk to someone.

Later that same evening, I am out on errands. Susan has gone to sleep. A quick trip, except as I walk out of the store, I pause. I wonder if the rabbi is still at the temple, which is not far from where we live—just under a mile. I decide to drop by and hope she is there. This evening is committee meeting night, and she probably is still there. I desperately need to talk to someone.

As I drive into the temple parking lot, I spy the rabbi's Subaru in her parking space. There are a few other cars scattered in the lot. She is here! Hopefully, she won't be on her way out the back door as I walk in the front door.

Indeed, as I enter the building, turn right and head down the hallway, I hear nothing. The temple feels as empty as my heart, which now begins to beat more rapidly. Anxious, I walk quickly around the hallway in the hexagon-shaped building looking for anyone. Where is everyone? I come around a corner and hear voices from the classroom area, where the last committee meeting is ending. I start to walk faster and almost bump into the rabbi, walking toward her office and me.

"Oh, hi, Sam," she says. "What brings you here so late?"

"Rabbi, I need to talk. Do you have a few minutes, please?"

I notice a slight facial sigh. I can tell the rabbi is tired and imagine her thought: *Oh shit, something else. Okay, I can do this.*

"Come into my office, Sam. Let's chat while I pack up my things if you don't mind. Joshua and the kids are waiting for me. I need to get home. Sorry, it's just so late."

A large desk faces the couch and two chairs. The rabbi walks around to the back of the desk, pulls up a small briefcase, and starts inserting some file folders from her desk. I sit down. She looks up, pausing for a second with that "well?" look, and so I start. Suddenly it's hard for me to talk. I mumble, "I need to talk about Susan."

Even before I get Susan's name out, she interrupts. "Oh, you're sad that Susan won't be around to see the grandkids grow up. And she won't be able to be at their bar and bat mitzvot?"

I freeze in place, barely able to breathe. The rabbi doesn't seem to notice the silence. She keeps packing up. Her eyes lift briefly, looking through me as if I'm not in the room. My silence doesn't seem to register with her.

Internally, I am screaming. "No. No. It is none of that! What I need to know is how am I going to do this? How am I going to dance the last, the actual dance with Susan?"

I can't, I know, really say any of this. The rabbi is already at the private door that leads from her study to the parking lot. She opens it, her hand inviting me to precede her. I walk her to her car. And I do thank her for her time. I do not, though, tell her about the voices, or the orchestra, or the ballroom.

The rabbi backs out of her reserved parking spot next to the building. She waves and smiles before speeding out onto the street. Now, alone in the temple's empty parking lot on this chilly spring night, disturbed, time once again goes to infinity.

I hear the orchestra practicing now. I am scared and confused by the sounds and smells and images, the sense of being here in this ballroom and somewhere else—now the parking lot of the temple—at the very same time. I hear the orchestra practicing more clearly by the hour. The orchestra is real and is everywhere.

The orchestra warming up sounds as vibrant as anything else in the so-called 'real world.' It exists, and it is everywhere! The sounds explode in my head— violins, cellos, basses, clarinets, French horns, flutes, piccolos, and even giant harps. They are as real as every other sound around me. I don't understand why other people don't hear them.

I need to talk to someone else. I wonder if the psychiatrist I have seen now and then for the past twenty years is still in practice. It has been about a decade since I last saw him. I look for his phone number in my Rolodex, and yes, the card with Dr. Goldstein's number is still there. Not surprising, since I never remove a card from my Rolodex, I just add to it—a personal quirk that lets me sometimes remember friends and colleagues I've lost.

I call the number to see if it might work. Not only does it work, but his office is still on the same floor and office suite that it had been during my last visit about a decade ago.

The first time I saw him, I was depressed as I struggled to succeed in my new role as a boss. I had never managed people before becoming the executive director of a small nonprofit. We started to grow after I came on board, adding staff, and soon I was out of my league. Employees complained about me to anyone who would listen. I lost confidence in myself and didn't know what to do about it. The time I spent with Dr. Goldstein back then helped tremendously, and I have been a massive fan of psychotherapy ever since.

Now that I am facing the worst crisis in my life, who better to see than Dr. Goldstein? I make an appointment. I must have expected the office suite to be the same as it was a decade earlier because I am disoriented when I walk back into this place. The waiting room is smaller than I remember, and their office decor has changed. There is now a glass partition separating the office staff from arriving patients. I wonder if they're currently involved in treating drug addiction.

Dr. Goldstein comes out and walks me into his office, which is much the same as it has always been. I sit down across from him for what will turn out to be our only session.

I tell him about Susan's breast cancer, and about the orchestra, and the ballroom, and the dance. I explain how real the ballroom is to me. Secretly, I am afraid I might be losing my mind. I wonder—no, I hope he will give me medication. He did that the last time I saw him. I think the medicine will remove the images, erase the orchestra, and change the future by changing what is going on in my head.

I say all of this through streaming tears. Almost sobbing!

He looks at me for a long moment, silent, just seemingly staring. I understand that this clinical, blank stare is because psychiatrists are not supposed to show reactions. "Why are you crying?" he asks in a flat voice.

The question surprises me. It seems evident to me. This passive-aggressive psychiatric crap gets to me, and I bark: "Susan's going to die! I am having these crazy visions. I don't know what is going on with me! I'm afraid I'm losing my mind!"

He doesn't react to my irritation. I notice his eyes are moist. He then breaks protocol and reacts to what I have said. "Sam, you bring a deep and moving dignity to such a terrible moment. It's beautiful."

CHAPTER 12

Wrestling

"Beauty. Dignity." Dr. Goldstein's simple words have a dramatic impact on me. It's as if a hood has slowly lifted off my head, and the world is different. I can breathe. I can see a different path to this inevitable end.

Rather than fearing this ultimate loss, this moment of grace taking place in a different dimension of time and space, I think I will be able to get ready for what I call The Actual Dance. I now understand that the actual dance will be the ultimate consummation of our love. That which I never wanted to do, never imagined I could, I now know I can. I will hold Susan in an ultimate embrace, graced with perfect comfort and perfect love, as she slowly dissolves from my embrace into that bright light.

As we prepare to have the lump removed and her condition reassessed, I remain buoyed by Dr. Goldstein's assurances during those brief moments in his office. I don't know if Susan can sense a change in me. I do not tell her about my session with Dr. Goldstein. I continue to hide these inexplicable experiences, fears, and terrors that consume me. She doesn't know about the ballroom nor the ritual that is now ingrained in my being. I still don't understand it, and I continue to suspect it may be a hallucination. But I don't care as much. Dr. Goldstein didn't offer me medicine to eliminate these moments of seeing the world from the outside, as if I am a traveling spirit. He didn't say it was a hallucination. Instead, he called it a metaphor and said that it is beautiful.

Twenty years earlier, when I first sought treatment with Dr. Goldstein for depression and anxiety, he told me he wished we could have had time for a full Freudian-style psychoanalysis. What were the core causes of my fears and behaviors? I wonder now if those subconscious demons are now in a world championship battle for my soul. The sessions back then changed me. They turned my life around. I knew then that I had more work to do and that other challenges would compel me to seek help in the future. Significant personal change is hard. There is no magic to this process. And, unfortunately, there is no magic to heal Susan.

Now the waiting begins again. We need to find out if, as everyone expects, the unexpected lump is an aggressive spread of breast cancer. I'm angry with myself for my momentary lapse, allowing myself to think that everything might just turn out relatively okay. I once again know full well how this will end. I have traveled this road before.

One grandfather, two grandmothers, four aunts, two uncles, Susan's father, my father, my sister, Susan's mother, and yes, my mother. Death has been a constant presence in my life for as long as I remember.

I was just five years old when a cacophony of voices in the house roused me at 7 a.m. Even at that age, I could sense something was wrong. As I stepped into a hallway, I saw my parents and older sisters heading out the door at the far end of a long hallway. "Where are you going?" I yelled.

Someone turned around and yelled back, "Grandpa Simon has died; we are heading to the house. We will be back as soon as we can."

I still remember watching as my parents disappeared down the steps to the driveway into the bright light of outside, their dark shadows silhouetted against the darkened hallway. That was the start of my life as a perpetual spiritual bystander.

In those days, Harding and Orr's Funeral Home offered a standard funeral package that included the casket, the funeral services, and transportation for the family in long black limousines. The funeral home occupied a converted, brown-brick mansion with a covered arched drive-thru entrance. Upon arrival, the funeral director would meet us and escort us to a private area reserved for the immediate family.

My memory is of a large room with brick walls, a soaring ceiling, and rows of pews. In the front was an extended platform just a single step above the floor. A speaker's stand on the left corner faced forward. There was also an organ and a place for a choir or just a soloist.

The routine is familiar. Each time the same, beginning with my mother's mother when I was just seven years old, then my mom's sisters Julia and Hunchy, and then Mom herself, my two uncles, and my sister Harriet. In the era of Green Stamps, I sometimes wondered if there were "Frequent Burial Points."

I believed I was an emotional bystander in those moments, observing my parents and aunts and uncles crying and reacting. I became encased with a thick emotional veneer that is now about to crack wide open. The ballroom is my sanctuary, relieving the pressure from the emotional tsunami that wants to engulf me. While I now recognize it as a gift of beauty and dignity—the ecstatic consummation of our love—I still fear the looming prospect of being alone, of infinite silence, of losing the other half of my whole. Despite the alternate universe I continue to experience, I live in the real world.

Right now, the real world is unfolding in the surgical center of Inova Fair Oaks Hospital. As calm and collected as I may seem on the outside, inside, I am down for the count, wrestling with God and losing. In one corner, I am the man in the tuxedo in the ballroom about to hold the love of my life in my arms as she takes her last breath. The ultimate gift for both of us, an ultimate goodbye. In the other corner, I am the man about to have half of his soul ripped out, which will end my life as I know it.

CHAPTER 13

The Moment Arrives

Susan's brother, Melvin, arrives on a Thursday afternoon. I fill him in on the chin-up attitude we need to have around Susan. We need to arrive at Fair Oaks Hospital by 7 a.m. on Friday for the procedure to remove the new lump.

The Fair Oaks Hospital experience is new for Susan and me. We have never been to this particular facility. The unfamiliarity adds to the emotional intensity of the moment, at least for me. Susan doesn't show any concern, and Melvin is quiet. We search for where to park. Out-patient surgery patients have their reserved spaces, but we don't know that and drive around in circles for a bit. A wall hides the door to the admissions desk; it takes us a moment to figure that out. All this confusion just raises the stakes of what already seems to me like a life-and-death moment.

Susan walks up to the check-in station at precisely seven o'clock, with Melvin and me right behind. Whew, we made it! The three of us take a breath and take a seat. A nurse comes right out to escort Susan to the pre-op area. I get up to go with them as I did for the mastectomy. This time though, I'm stopped and sent back to the waiting room to sit with Melvin. I interpret not being allowed to wait with Susan in the pre-op bay as ominous. While my being banished to the waiting room probably just has to do with the procedure being deemed minor and routine, it's anything but minor and routine to us. Dr. Happy will remove the lump and, if necessary, send it off for analysis. If the lump is, as everyone expects, cancer, Susan's prognosis is grim.

As I head back to sit next to Melvin, my eyes scan this large, dimly lit waiting room, empty, except for Melvin and me. The magnitude of the moment overwhelms me, and in mid-stride, I disappear into the ballroom.

I stand at the edge of the blond wood dance floor. People are now gathering around the darkened back of the ballroom. They add a constant murmur to the background. I gaze into that mass of people, sensing them rather than seeing anyone. I know who they are—everyone Susan and I have ever met, ever known, or ever loved in our lives. Not only have our children and family and friends come for this moment, but even generations of family who came before us are in attendance. As I circle along the edges of the ballroom dance floor, I wonder if crunched around these darkened walls aren't also generations yet to come. Eternity—no beginning—no end.

The orchestra is playing now. At first, I can barely make out the tune. Then I hear it! "Unchained Melody," our song. We fell in love with it the first time we saw the movie Ghost.

I don't think anyone else recognizes the tune, but I do, and I know that Susan will. She will love it.

I step out into the center of the dance floor. I am dressed comfortably, with a perfectly fitting tuxedo. Vest. Bow tie. I am expecting Susan, having donned an elegant gown, to join me at any moment. She appears suddenly, manifesting from nothing into a glowing, angelic emanation seemingly floating toward me.

Suddenly, the very last scene of the movie Ghost pops into my head. I believe in ghosts. I do. I can hear in my head the very last words in that movie—"the love inside of you, you take it with you"—because I think they will be Susan and my last words to each other.

And then I'm back, somehow seated next to Melvin, his face still deep in a newspaper, unaware that I left his side. I wonder how long I was gone. Time in the ballroom, I have come to accept, is different than in the real world.

We wait. I fidget. Someone else enters the waiting area and sits far away from us. The silence and anticipation continue until Dr. Happy casually steps out of a door still in his operating room garb. Melvin and I look up at him and then each other. Should Melvin go up with me to hear the news? No, I am the only one who can do this. It is my responsibility and mine alone. The ultimate act of love that I prayed I would never have to do, that I was afraid to do, and that I have come to know I have to do. *This is how we will consummate our love.* I remind myself, *I am the other half of her whole. I can do this.*

The orchestra is playing now. In a classic waltz pose, I stand in the dance floor center, expecting Susan's essence, which entered the ballroom, to now join me. I wait, and the

music becomes loud, and the crowd does not move. Then the
music becomes even louder and the moment more intense. I
expect Susan to join me any instant now.

Then, everything stops before Susan has joined me. I no
longer see her at all. Just silence now.

The musicians stand, pack up their instruments, and get
ready to leave. I slowly turn and notice that the perimeter of
the ballroom is empty now. The lights start to come up ever so
slightly. I am still standing there, alone, in the center of the
dance floor, when each orchestra member exits past me, just
as they entered in front of me—not acknowledging me, not
reacting in any way, seemingly off to their next assignment.

And Susan and I have not danced the actual dance.

"It's not cancer, Sam. It's not cancer! Dr. Happy's
ebullient voice brings me back into the here and now. He
puts his hand on my left shoulder. "It's just a plain old
water cyst." His voice is almost cracking.

Incredulous, I look over at Melvin, who is still staring
at me. I wonder if I made a mistake having him come up
from Houston. I give a thumbs-up and smile.

Just as I start to walk over to him, Susan, fully dressed,
struts out of the same door from which Dr. Happy had
emerged. "Let's go home, Sam, Melvin." She seems to
have expected the news—or willed it into being.

As I drive Susan and Melvin home, my eyes see not
the road ahead but instead the inside of a now empty
grand ballroom where only moments before the actual
dance was in full production.

The ballroom sits silent, semi-dark, empty. I am the only one here, the orchestra off to play somewhere else. A different favorite tune for another couple, perhaps as they engage in a moment of grace. But for how long? How long until a new, different orchestra appears and invites Susan and me onto the dance floor as they play "Unchained Melody?"

Our next visit with Dr. Blonder, the oncologist, comes shortly after the procedure. Like the rest of the staff, the nurse, who knows us by now, invites Susan and me into the exam room with Dr. Blonder. He finds no unexpected lumps this time. No about-face turns to call anyone. Once again, Susan sheds her blouse to let a casual Dr. Blonder examine the scar-defined, silicon-implanted chest. The red areas around the incision lines are lighter, except where they took out that water cyst. Dr. Blonder again touches Susan's bare chest. His finger slides along the now barely visible scar from the original surgery. He stops at the freshly stitched area of the last biopsy. No problems.

Back in his office, he makes sure we recognize that the road forward is not simple. "Susan's prognosis is still highly guarded," he explains. He maps out sixteen weeks of aggressive chemotherapy and then six weeks of radiation treatments. Given the calendar and Susan's situation, he recommends starting the chemotherapy in a few weeks. The treatments will continue through the fall. She'll get a month or so off after chemotherapy before beginning radiation treatments in early 2001.

CHAPTER 14

Seeking a New Normal

*M*y job now is to create a sense of normalcy predicated on the pretense that this period is just a bump in the road of life and that we'll get through it together. Reluctantly, I go to the office every day, leaving Susan to recover from the mastectomy alone at home with our two dogs. My passion for work, leading a company I started fifteen years earlier that is now highly successful, has waned over these months. I notice but don't understand. Perhaps I am just exhausted from the pressure of Susan's illness.

The core of the company I founded in 1986, Issue Dynamics, Inc., revolves around my passion for social justice and changing the world. I am proud of our accomplishments. We are a leader in new forms of coalition building. We bring together for-profit companies and various nonprofit groups and unions to take technology to public schools in low-income communities. Until now, I have loved every minute of the journey. I can walk around downtown Washington, DC, from one client to the next who are just blocks apart. Now, going into the office feels like I am doing something wrong. It takes me away from where I'm supposed to be, taking care of Susan.

Conversely, Susan is ready to jump into where she left off. Shortly before her diagnosis, Susan and a friend had started a new business called Elder Affairs, an advisory service to help people deal with aging parents. She can't wait to get back to work. Her real job, of course, is to regain enough strength to start the chemotherapy. I detect an urgency in Dr. Blonder's desire to begin the treatment process as soon as possible. Susan doesn't seem to notice. She has a plan. She and her partner in Elder Affairs will divide up their work during her treatment. Susan will work the phones from home; her partner will do the in-person work with clients.

The first step involves another quick visit to the hospital's outpatient clinic for an infusion port to be inserted into Susan's upper left chest. The port, I learn, allows for a more rapid and direct infusion of chemotherapy's chemicals in a central vein. The medical staff can also draw blood through the port. It spares Susan and the nurses the challenge of finding solid veins in her arm every week.

I am more nervous than Susan as we get ready for her first chemotherapy session. I don't know what to expect. I've heard about the possible aftereffects of vomiting and fever, and the like. Apart from the infusion port, I just have no idea how the medical team administers the chemotherapy nor the role I will play in the process. Will I once again be sitting in a waiting room anticipating the worst?

Dr. Blonder offers Susan the option to be infused at Invoa Hospital's infusion center, or at the infusion center at their practice. It turns out that his extensive oncology practice has an infusion center in the same building as the oncology practice. It isn't clear to me why the location matters. I am a bit suspicious that his preference for his practice's center revolves around money. It doesn't take long into Susan's first chemo treatment at his practice for me to understand his preference for the infusion center in his office facility. He wants to be present.

Susan and I are both a bit anxious, or at least I am, as we head for Susan's first treatment and get lost finding the infusion center. It takes a few seconds to figure everything out. When we finally walk into a narrow entry area, the nurses greet Susan. They know her. Although the staff acknowledges me, I'm the odd man out.

We sit across from the nurse's station until someone comes to take us into the infusion area. We move tentatively into and then through the vast room with about a dozen infusion stations, each equipped with an oversize brown leather lounge chair, one or two IV stands, and a small table. We notice stacks of folding chairs available for added guests at each station line the back walls. The open room reminds me of the outpatient center full of people seated next to their loved ones where Susan had that first breast biopsy earlier this year.

Today only half the infusion stations are occupied. I see one man in a chair getting treatment. All the other patients are women. I am astonished that only half of the patients have a person sitting with them. *How can that be? How do they get home? Aren't they scared? What if they need something? What if something happens?*

I scan the room for the infusion station set up for Susan. I expect to see the IV already bagged, perhaps a nurse standing by, and even a chair set out for me. Instead, we just keep walking past it all and enter a short hallway. I'm confused. We make a broad U-turn and find ourselves in front of two private rooms. I immediately get it. Susan's infusion has risk associated with it, and she needs to be segregated—out of sight—in case something goes wrong. A silent confirmation of my worst fears.

Doctor Blonder and a second nurse appear and escort us into the small, private room on the right. Doctor Blonder, Susan, two nurses and I, crowd into what could be just a large closet in someone's home. I sit in a chair as Susan climbs onto what looks like a large table with pillows and blankets placed in advance on the right-back corner of the table.

We spend the first half-hour listening to Dr. Blonder explain the details of the chemotherapy regimen. It becomes clear that what they call a medical "cocktail" cre-ated to kill the cancer cells in Susan's body is the most potent treatment currently allowed by the Federal Drug Administration. Doctor Blonder explains that the drug combination is relatively new, and he wants Susan infused at the highest dosage allowed.

You don't have to beat me over the head to remind me that Susan's prognosis is poor. Just explain that she will be receiving a new treatment at the highest dosage allowed by the government. Susan hears this as good news. She is getting the latest and best option to make sure she survives.

I reflect on the earlier debate about where to do the infusion. Given the drugs' high dosage, should we be near the hospital's extensive medical capacity if something should go wrong? According to Doctor Blonder, infusing here has advantages because their unit is smaller, with more medical staff per patient than the hospital. Plus, these offices are within a mile of the hospital in the unlikely event something happens, and she needs to go to the ER.

Susan is ready to get started. I realize now that Susan's chemo will be administered through the port in the chest and that the other patients in the open room had the IV in their arms. Not a problem. Let's get going. She lies down on the table in her street clothes, not a gown, though her blouse is wide open to access the port. The nurse points out the blanket at the foot of the bed if she gets cold. A vomit bag sits nearby in case she gets sick. I sit back and watch, leaving my computer and fancy little Metricom modem in my briefcase. Nothing is routine this first time.

The nurses keep asking Susan how she feels. "It feels icy as it enters my chest, and I can feel the liquid spreading through my veins," she says.

"Are you nauseous?" I ask. She shakes her head, no. When Susan closes her eyes for a few minutes, I get nervous, though the nurse smiles at me. Slowly the bag empties, and Susan is done!

The staff tells us to wait for a half-hour to see if Susan will react to the drugs. This wait will be part of the routine throughout Susan's chemotherapy. Susan just sits and thumbs through magazines left in the room. She feels fine! Despite this first infusion's dramatic nature—separate back room, with both doctor and nurse—Susan's stoicism prevails. She never complains.

I am a novice at cancer. Maybe I should have prepared for the chemotherapy process by reading a book or joining a support group. Perhaps I should seek out other men going through this same process. Maybe, but I don't. Instead, I am present with Susan as much as possible. If I could will Susan's survival, it would be simple. Instead, thoughts of losing her, how I will handle that moment, and what I can do to avoid that moment continue to permeate my being and keep me in a state of high anxiety.

Unlike any other period in my life, I wrestle with who I am and what I am supposed to be. For nearly twenty-five years, from my early sessions back in 1980 with Dr. Goldstein, to slowly becoming a leader in my field, I've received significant recognition and experienced enormous pride in my children and family. Now I walk deep in the valley of the shadow of loss.

Who am I? What am I supposed to be? Where am I supposed to be?

The journey, however it ends, will be profound. Susan will require the support and love of as many people as possible. I know I should not try to do this alone. Yet, I cannot reveal to anyone what I know in my soul about how this story will end.

What seems like a new normal becomes a blur. March to June speed by so fast I barely remember a thing. The pre-chemo days were a deception, a trick to make me think we could find normal. Instead, everything in our life has changed, inside and out.

I ache all over, body and soul, as I grapple with competing emotions and a lack of vision of the future. The good news is that I no longer experience semi-blackout sessions in a grand empty ballroom. The bad news is I remain in a state of constant expectancy. *Is that them playing?* I wonder over and over and over again, expecting to be called back into the ballroom at any instant.

CHAPTER 15

Bumps in the Road

The first bump in the chemotherapy road comes on Saturday night following a Thursday chemo session, Susan's second. All during the day Saturday, Susan has felt weak and nauseous. Once again, I'm doing those things I thought I could never do. Help her get to the bathroom to be sick to her stomach. Help her climb back into bed. Take her temperature. By early evening she spikes a fever. At first, just 100. Still, we call Doctor Blonder on his nightline and let him know about the temperature and nausea. The service gets back to us within the hour to tell us the doctor wants us to monitor her for now, but if the temperature hits 103, we should go to the emergency room.

At 9 p.m., we retake her temperature. It has jumped to 104. Susan is woozy and finally agrees to go to the ER to get checked out. We alert Dr. Blonder's night service that we are heading to the ER. We know she might have to stay overnight, so we pack a bag of toiletries and nightclothes. Doctor Blonder has his office alert the hospital to expect us.

As usual, Susan remains calm while I anxiously focus on getting to the hospital as fast as possible. I don't know what to expect, so I fret. It has been a long time since we were last at Inova Fairfax's ER, and it was not a good experience. I had a high fever, yet the wait was so long we just walked out.

This time, the ER staff admits us upon arrival. They have Susan's entire medical history, including the details of her latest chemotherapy. They know she is highly immunocompromised. They have a private room set up for her. They take her temperature, and it is 105 degrees.

After a short debate about placing her in an ice bath, the nurses start an IV to get more fluids in her. They use the port. There is no obvious infection source right now, so the doctors will have to figure it out while in the hospital. Yes, they are going to keep her at least overnight. It takes only a few more minutes for a nurse to show up, and we all head back to the seventh floor. Familiar faces greet us. The nursing staff isn't surprised and tries to reassure me, I think, more than Susan. "This happens all the time," they say.

I learn a lot about oncology nursing. I had not realized that oncology nurses are the elite of nursing, along with the ICU nurses. During this visit, I notice things about the nurses I didn't the last visit. They effuse purpose and gentleness. They never show fear or lack of confidence.

They are efficient, sometimes in a hurry, and yet not at the expense of noticing everyone.

Nurses pop into the room now whenever they are on duty to just check in on both of us. "Why are you back?" two different ones ask. I mention Susan's fever, and they both immediately reassure me that everything will be fine. "It happens all the time, don't worry."

Susan is irritated with my fawning over her. She is insistent that she is going to be okay. "Stay home, Sam," she demands, noting that I didn't think to bring nightclothes or toiletries for myself. "You're making me nervous. Besides, who is going to take care of Lucky and Maddie?" Reluctantly, I go home to be with the dogs, who sense that something is wrong. They do not bark when I walk into an otherwise empty house at 2 a.m., though they seem to wait expectantly for Susan to walk in behind me.

I sit alone for a time in the empty family room on a couch in a silence that empties my soul. "Is this how life is, being alone?" My mind wants to hide from the thought that won't hide. I am in a place that Dr. Goldstein didn't tell me exists. It is the other, darker angel in my struggle. The ledge of a chasm of a never-ending plunge into the place I fear most.

Good news. The following day Susan's fever has dropped. The doctor says Susan should stay one or two more days just to make sure the antibiotic works. We are reminded again by Dr. Blonder of Susan's high-risk profile and that the chemo drugs she is getting are the most powerful on the market today.

Following this infection and three days in the hospital, Dr. Blonder decides to add a new medicine to increase her immunity—an injection of medication to boost her white blood cell count. It isn't unusual in chemotherapy for patients to take medicine to improve their immunity to infections. The drug must be injected into her thigh area, something that Susan and I will learn to do. Whenever possible, I administer the shot, in part because I am more adept at this than Susan and because I find it hard to imagine forcing Susan to inject herself.

Giving my wife a shot in the thigh is, incredibly, an act of love. I discover that I can do things I never thought possible and which creates a deep intimacy. Feeling, touching, and noticing are now different from before. The worst moments in the hospital, those that sent me into the ballroom of anticipation, were different. Now, injecting her in her thigh, I am engulfed with oneness with her in our home. It fills a deep well of fear with more and more love.

It only takes a few more weeks into the chemotherapy for Susan's hair to begin to fall out. Wig shopping is followed by the ritual haircut and shaving off all the rest of her hair.

Even now, deep in the post-mastectomy treatment world, Susan and I continue to exist on separate planes of this universe. On her plane, despite the surgery, her bald head, nausea, exhaustion, lymphedema (localized swelling), and a highly guarded prognosis, everything is going to be "just fine." She projects warmth and confidence throughout the process. Her North Star continues to be the title of Gloria Gainer's "I Will Survive." Her approach echoes Bubbie Roz's, "Everything is going to be just fine."

On my plane? I continue to wait and listen. I have figured out what that other place is, what I now just refer to as "the ballroom." I can now will myself there. I just take a breath, close my eyes, and leave the here and now for the peace and grace of a different dimension of time and space, where I stand alone, listening for an orchestra and preparing for the inevitable last chapter in our story. Nonetheless, if the ballroom is a way station to the divine, life without Susan still looms as an abyss. I fight to stay clear of it.

Once again, tension develops between Susan and me over my desire to be with her at every moment. She wants our life to return to some form of pre-cancer normality. "Sam, I don't need you to babysit me! I am going to be just fine." I often hear it in different ways, sometimes through exasperated words, other times through short silent treatments, or in her demeanor as she pushes me away. I already know there will never again be a *before*. Everything is now different. Even so, I get the message. She can keep herself busy. Word about her cancer has spread widely; neighbors, friends, and family are not far if she has a crisis.

In the middle of Susan's aggressive chemotherapy treatments, we get a VIP invitation to the August 2000

Democratic National Convention in California. And because most of the Simon family—Susan, our son, and I—are active in the Virginia Democratic Party, we will also be part of the state's delegation as non-voting delegates with VIP access. We might even meet the next president if we go.

I am delighted, indeed feeling a bit like a hotshot. I want to accept the invitation, except Susan has advanced breast cancer and is in the middle of a new, aggressive chemotherapy regimen. She's been in and out of the hospital now twice—the ER, a private holding room, and back to the seventh floor for a day or two. Going to the convention across the country doesn't seem feasible nor wise.

Strangely, Susan's medical team encourages us to make the trip.

"What an exciting opportunity! You guys should go. It will take some effort, but you can make it work. First, we need to make sure your immune system is strong enough to avoid infections. Sam, you will need to give Susan an immunity booster shot. It is similar to what we gave her after the first infection, but stronger." The difference, too, is that this more potent medicine needs to be injected into her stomach.

As a further safety measure, the oncologist will arrange for Susan to be seen and tested midweek at Cedars Sinai hospital's outpatient cancer center clinic. They will do blood tests and give us additional medication.

I read between the lines. Doctor Blonder's and Doctor Morgan's matter-of-fact assurances that we can make the proposed trip feasible means they don't expect Susan to survive. They understand this will be a once in a very brief remaining lifetime opportunity for Susan.

Susan and I both have reservations. The moment is a bit like the conversation moment after finding out the cancer was in Susan's lymph nodes—what should we do with the precious little time left in our lives? Instead of a conversation, this time, our decision-making unfolds in real time. With a clearer sense of what might happen to her, the opportunity feels a little bit like taking that trip around the world while still living the life we love to live. Besides, I have cousins in LA who we can see and reach out to for help if we need it.

Susan isn't sure and suggests I go myself. "It's just a work thing, Sam. I might be in your way."

I need to nudge Susan into her *yes*. "Look, Susan, even the doctors are encouraging us to go. It will be good for your spirits."

In retrospect, this trip seems to have been absurd. Who the hell would think this is a good idea? Yet, the Los Angeles trip goes amazingly well. Our Congressman dotes on Susan and introduces both of us to all the right people. The Democrats nominate Al Gore and Joe Lieberman at this convention. Later Susan and I will host Joe Lieberman at our home for a fundraiser.

This risky trip's success forges a path to new confidence. Susan finishes her chemotherapy treatments a month later. No more late-night ER visits. The next step is radiation treatments that won't start until after the first of the year. This break in Susan's treatment comes just in time for her fifty-fifth Birthday, October 25th, 2000—her first birthday as a breast cancer survivor. We celebrate, hosting a big party with friends and family at our home.

That night, we extend the celebration by having sex, our first since the mastectomy. Not that we haven't seen each other naked or anything like that. We have just held each other and have been intimate in different ways. On this evening, we carefully navigate each other's bodies. In bed together, Susan, still wearing a small sports halter to cover her scarred chest, snuggles. "Let's do this more often!"

I wrap my arm around her, feeling the warmth of her touch on the outside. Inside, a cavernous emptiness echoes in my soul, sensing this too may never happen again. I feel as alone at this moment with Susan in my arms as I did as I sat by myself in the waiting room of Hermann Hospital in 1967. "Yes, more often," I whisper, trying to hold back tears. I think about what to say if she asks me why I'm crying.

As 2000 ends, Susan's energy and strength grow. Our routine in life approaches near post-breast cancer normality. At least for a few months. In January 2001, the oncologist clears her to see the radiologist. The radiologist and the oncologist agree—Susan needs to get the maximum radiology routine.

I am not surprised. Nothing has changed for me. I still carry the burden of a deep knowing that despite the optimism of any given moment, Susan's illness is going to win. Cancer beat her mother and destroyed mine. I cannot shake the belief that it will beat her, too. I don't know how and I don't know when. I just know it is inevitable. Yes, I try to talk myself out of these thoughts and pretend from time to time that I'm wrong. These tricks don't work. I know the truth.

During our first visit, the head of radiology at Fairfax Inova Hospital explains the process and the likely side effects—redness or a burning sensation in the target areas and perhaps some fatigue. Susan's treatment schedule will start in February.

Radiation is radically different from chemotherapy, so I am not in the room with the big machines during her first radiation treatment. Susan goes back with a nurse to the radiology machines and returns fifteen minutes later dressed and ready to go as if nothing happened.

"Most people drive themselves to treatments," the radiologist tells us.

Susan, it turns out, can do this without my help. She settles into the treatment routine with negligible impact on either of us. Increasingly, our life routine feels almost normal, except for her periodic trips to have radiation therapy. Indeed, I continue to fret silently over when her cancer will return, for I know it will. I live my life with that certainty. I still do everything I can to hide this from Susan, even as life seems to return to a new normal.

The next chapter in this saga could be titled "The Hair." Susan's hair is growing back, causing her wig to feel tight and itchy. She takes it off whenever she is not in public, revealing a stubble that has emerged bright white. Technically, I guess it's gray, but it looks white. Her two brothers, Melvin and Buddy, have hair that is bright white/gray. While I suspect her brothers' hair was somewhat darker when Susan and I were first married, I only remember them with white hair. Susan, on the other hand, has been coloring her hair black for nearly thirty years now.

But now what? Should she dye her hair again or leave it natural? I vote for dye. Susan disagrees. "Let's leave it natural, Sam." As it grows back, the translucent white hair imparts a new elegance to Susan that everyone, including me, notices. Increasingly smart- and professional-looking, she projects a new persona.

Susan's radiation treatments are a snap compared to the chemotherapy. Just as the radiologist had warned us, the worst side effects are fatigue and burning, and tenderness at the site.

Her active treatments end as spring of 2001 is turning to summer. Susan has gone through the standard of care: A double mastectomy, chemotherapy, and radiation. Check, check, check. We start the five-year clock of watchful waiting. The medical community maintains that if a treated cancer does not recur within five years, the patient is "cured." Any cancer after that is deemed new or different. I, of course, know better. My mother's breast cancer reappeared seven years after she finished treatment, and no one doubts it was her breast cancer waking up. My doctor was right when he told me that the cancer cells spread throughout a body long before cancer became detectable in the body.

On October 25th of 2001, Susan turns fifty-six. We both clearly remember the day in 1967 when her mom took her last breath at fifty-six years old. This year, as we enter the post-treatment era, I have zero confidence that the quarterly checkups will be routine. I expect a metastasis. Susan knows the significance of getting through the year and of outliving her mother. She is more determined than ever to stay cancer-free.

The checkup process is easy compared to previous treatments. A nurse takes blood for analysis, and Dr. Blonder performs a physical exam to make sure no new lumps have appeared anywhere. I am not in the room. I don't need to keep watching another man put his hands all over Susan's body. I join Dr. Blonder and Susan in his office to review all the results.

I stare as Dr. Blonder talks to Susan to see if I can discern a subtext in his words. I still remember the moment during the first exam when he did his military-style about-face. Thankfully, his words and body gestures all remain positive. "Good news, Susan. You are clear for now." I sigh silently inside when he adds, "Let's hope this keeps up."

Then I jump in.

"Great, Dr. Blonder! Can she take anything to reduce the likelihood of recurrence and spread?"

"No, not yet, Sam. Hopefully soon."

Dr. Blonder and I develop a rapport. I feel his empathy, his energy to keep Susan healthy, and his desire to be hopeful. I think he respects me and my determination to find something new and different to help Susan. On the other hand, perhaps he has tired of answering my frequent questions about new treatments because he comes up with a plan for me.

CHAPTER 16

Changing the Future

"Expect an invitation to join the Community Cancer Advisory Committee," Dr. Blonder tells me.

The committee is an Inova Fairfax hospital initiative to increase Inova's ratings in the *U.S. News and World Report* rankings of cancer hospitals. It's also a way for me to gain insights into the future. Indeed, each time Inova Cancer Center hosts a lecture or a seminar for the medical staff about the latest treatments in breast cancer, as a committee member, I get invited. Two years into this routine, while attending a lecture about new therapies, I raise my hand for the first time to ask a question in a room filled with doctors. When I inquire about patients like Susan who have what will become known as triple-negative chemistry, I receive the same response I've gotten for the last seven years. "No. I'm sorry, still no known treatments or medicine."

Even though I seek a miracle, I expect that answer. Of course, I don't articulate any of this to Susan, who is perfectly happy with her current medical team and treatments. She isn't looking for miracles. She expects everything to be just fine.

I spend much of my spare time scouring medical publications for information about treatments and break-through medicines for Susan's condition. I learn that metastasis can show up anywhere, though most often in the bone, liver, lungs, or brain. My mother's cancer metas-tasized to her brain, so I focus on that. Every time Susan gets a headache, I worry. Since Susan also has a sensitive stomach and is allergic to all sorts of foods, I also catastro-phize almost daily the slightest stomach problem.

This post-treatment world is full of positive surprises for Susan, starting with her new and unexpected deep commitment to exercise. She begins by taking stretch classes and then gets more serious. When she returns to work, she gets up early every morning and heads to the gym for an hour of exercise before heading to work. Her commitment to complete recovery shows in her increasingly athletic body. In addition to exercising, she eats a healthy diet and, as always, maintains a positive attitude. These habits, I read in health journals, are the activities that best predict longevity. She does them intuitively.

I fall into silent depression. I don't exercise with Susan. Instead, I just get up, shower, and head into the commute to Washington, DC, to engage in a rote work-life because I don't know what else to do. As traffic from McLean to

Washington, DC, a mere ten miles, intensifies every year, I try to beat the worst of rush hour by getting up and leaving earlier and earlier every morning. At one time, I could leave the house at 7:30 a.m.; I now have to head in between 6:45 and 7:00. As the boss, I always felt the need to be the first person in the office and usually the last to leave. Now I just do it because that's what I've always done.

Traffic isn't my only excuse for not going to the gym with Susan. I have gained nearly forty-five pounds over the last eighteen months. My weight when Susan was first diagnosed at the start of 2000 was around 199. Now, I am about 245 pounds. I am obese. It has taken me less than a year to grow into double extra-large and the Big Men sections of clothing stores.

When Susan and I married, I was skinny—130 pounds at 6' 2" tall. No wonder some folks called me *String Bean* and *Spaghetti Sam*. I was always a heavy smoker, up to three packs a day, which is probably what kept me so thin. I finally entered a program called *Smokenders*—the most challenging task in my entire life, until now. It took six months to stop and years to overcome the desire to go back. Of course, I compensated. Over the next five years as a nonsmoker, I ate compulsively and gained fifteen pounds a year until I topped off around 240 pounds. It took me attending Weight Watchers with Susan in the late 1990s to get back to what I consider my fighting weight of 199 pounds. Then the cancer journey started, and our Weight Watchers discipline disappeared. Susan wasn't well enough to go for nearly a year. I just fell off the proverbial wagon. The emotional stress of what I call the era of active waiting and watching does not help.

As time goes by, with all of Susan's exercise and seeming normality, my apprehension ebbs, and I slip into thinking perhaps we have entered a new, post-cancer, everything-is-fine world. Still, Susan's health regime seems homeopathic. Exercise, diet, and the right attitude are not medicine. So, while I recognize that healthy living styles and general health are adding to years of survival, I continue to hunt for new medical advances that will reduce the likelihood of recurrence of her triple-negative breast cancer.

Despite what everyone else now sees as a happy ending, and my occasional lapses into hope, I do not change. The years do not matter. I continue to be an emotional pasta bowl when it comes to Susan. Deeply seeded within my soul rests an inner truth that twists and twirls and rattles my core—the perfect knowledge that something is wrong. I have neither the language nor the capacity to name *it*, this apparent ability to see the future with some form of a gift—or curse. Can I see things that no other person can see? Yes. I saw my mother's soul exit her at her last breath. Of course, I can know my wife's ultimate destiny. I just can't tell anyone these things.

I will come to understand that I struggle with a consequence of anticipatory grief I have since named Post-Traumatic Spiritual Disorder—the psychological stress associated with my anticipation of holding Susan as she takes her last breath. I imagine this is not different from the post-traumatic stress disorder experienced by the soldier involved in trauma who believes it's over. Then one day, a car backfires, and the mind again explodes with images and smells.

While Susan lives now solidly in a post-cancer era, my life is a series of confirmations of just the opposite. Each time Susan complains of an ache or pain, I listen. I wonder. News like "no new drugs" or hearing of another death triggers me. Each time, I listen for that orchestra waiting to enter an empty grand ballroom, hovering in that time and space of an alternative dimension. At the *yahrzeit*—anniversary—of my mother's death or Susan's mother, I listen. Just sitting in the temple as the rabbi reads the names out loud, I can take Susan's hand and suddenly enter that different zone of the universe. I look down from above as I stand in the center of an empty, grand ballroom, seeing us—Susan, me—together perhaps for the last time.

I don't understand what's happening to me. Soldiers with stress disorders from the trauma of war tend to relive those moments of pain and loss, yet most are on a healing journey. My trauma continues unabated, with each figurative "and just one more thing," adding to the distress. I don't have anything to get over; it has not happened yet.

CHAPTER 17

Signs and Omens

*W*ill I ever really believe that everything is going to be "just fine?" Is there a time limit on this disease— this spiritual disorder? I know that her body is full of sleeping cancer cells that lie inert, just waiting for something to turn them on and then suffocate her. Will my cure come when I believe a new drug or treatment or other good news from somewhere predicts longevity for people like Susan? I hope so.

Until then, life remains this wrestling match, a series of up-and-down, in-and-out, almost-there-and-back-again challenges. I look for signs and omens to help me move from the ballroom to "just fine." I need a small peg on which to hang a thin veneer of hope again. The universe, it seems, conspires to send just the opposite messages.

Although our lives' growing routine creates a façade of normality, what might have been a path to "just fine" is brutally interrupted by what I call *Joan's journey*.

Joan is the same Joan who recommended her oncologist to us. The one we met with before selecting Dr. Blonder. She is also part of the temple's breast cancer support group. Her husband, Stan, is Susan's dentist, and both are active members of the temple.

Joan and Stan have kept in close touch throughout Susan's breast cancer treatment phase. We learn that Joan is now pessimistic about her prognosis. Stan calls to invite us to dinner at their beautiful home. It becomes clear that we are part of his plan to support Joan. As we dine, he invites us to join them for a weekend at their beach house in Bethany Beach, Maryland. It seems that Stan is hoping to expose Joan to Susan's positive outlook.

The beach weekend allows us to know our hosts a little too well. Joan and Stan bicker most of the time, and we see Joan's pessimism firsthand. Rather than trying to "fix" Joan, Susan won't have any of it. She has spent years now refusing to allow negativity into her life. The shield she carries to guard against pessimism, the barrier I still see, isn't going to crack. There is no door nor window through which someone else who might need help will be allowed to enter. The risk to herself is too high. We spend most of our time on the beach alone, and after the weekend, we politely keep our distance.

Despite our best efforts, Joan and Stan continue to intrude into our lives. Our paths cross at an improbable rate and in circumstances that convince us that some higher force is at work.

Just one year later, Susan and I run into Stan and Joan in the middle of the Festival Fringe in Edinburgh, Scotland. Yes, run into them. Susan and I are sitting at a table at an outdoor cafe on a random day in August, in the middle of Edinburgh, Scotland, amongst a crowd of thousands of people, when Susan spots Joan and Stan.

It is worth repeating. On our first vacation since Susan's mastectomy, we made our first trip to Scotland, as it happens, during the Edinburgh Festival Fringe. With hundreds of thousands of people in attendance, Joan and Stan suddenly appear in the middle of the main street, and Susan sees them! What are the odds? It's as if the universe is telling us: "Pay attention." The question becomes why.

When Joan and Stan see Susan waving, they run over, sit down, and we all go on about the coincidence of running into each other. How the hell can this be? We are still conscious of not being too close to them back at the temple, yet they are now at our table. Something is wrong with this situation. My mind tells me that Susan and Joan share some sort of fate. It wakes up the ballroom and scares the hell out of me.

It gets more bizarre. We see them again the next night at a restaurant. We have reservations at the same place, at the same time for dinner in Edinburgh, Scotland. Of course. Why not?

A tug of war explodes inside my soul with each of these inexplicable events. Susan experiences them as good fun and perhaps a way to help Joan; I see them telling me what lies ahead for us.

Notwithstanding running into Joan and Stan, this trip to Scotland is crucial to our, Susan's and Sam's, desire to find a new normal, a normal that includes more time together. When Susan and I sat down in the spring of 2000 to have "the conversation," our focus was on the external part of our lives—jobs, possessions, travel. Now we seek a more meaningful life with each other.

Having gained the confidence to travel in the post-treatment world, upon our return from Scotland, we immediately look ahead to another trip for the end of December 2001. We love the sun, and the beach as winter starts at home, and over the decades have made spending December on a Caribbean Island a tradition. Excited to make up for the last two years we missed and buoyed by Edinburgh, we look for something different and pick Cabo San Lucas in Mexico. We base our choice on the memorable trip our son and his wife had there this past summer.

We are nervous and excited to arrive at a brand-new resort city in December of 2001. As we usually do on our first full day in a country on these trips, we take a bus tour to get our bearings. Our bus pulls into an overlook, high above the city.

"There's Stan!" Susan screams as she steps off the bus. And then, "There's Joan."

Really. Stan and Joan are not only in Cabo: they are also on a bus tour that simultaneously comes to the same stop as our bus tour. Another "coincidence?"

The moment is brutal for me. I am spooked already by what happened in Edinburgh. Now, again in Cabo, the most unlikely coincidence ever, once again, Stan and Joan. Sam and Susan. I am confused and afraid. I want to open my mind, clear it from rational thinking, and allow the ineffable, who has made this happen, to enable me to understand why. I am convinced that these two encounters can't be random. I know, as much as I know anything else to be true, that our lives are interconnected for a reason or a purpose. What is it?

The universe answers in the fall of 2003 when we learn that Joan's breast cancer has returned. She dies a few months later. At the funeral in our temple sanctuary, I stand back as Susan and all the other women from the temple's breast cancer support group encircle the casket, hold hands, and sing a Debbie Friedman song of goodbye. Susan is crying. My stomach is in my throat.

Looking down from above, staring at this incredible moment of a casket surrounded by Jewish women, hand in hand, singing, I transform, once again away, no longer in the temple.

I am standing at the center of the dance floor of a faintly illuminated ballroom. Movement is now discernable in the unlit back of the ballroom. Are those musicians, or are they just our ancestors from generations past moving up to take their places? These disturbing images come in and out of my mental vision.

Upon my return to awareness in the sanctuary, I stand on the temple bema (the elevated platform) above the casket and watch the women, Susan among them, sway and sing as they hold hands. This moment is a rehearsal for what is coming. I can see the upcoming moment of women gathered around Susan's casket, the breast cancer group singing Debbie Friedman songs. What else could this mean?

I imagine what I would say—or if I would be able to say anything—at Susan's funeral. I recall being at the funeral of my cousin, who the rabbi called "truly a woman of valor," and Susan telling me then, "I hope that they can say that about me. I want to be known as a woman of valor."

Now, years later, as I look at Joan's casket and see it instead as Susan's, I know that the first line of my eulogy for Susan will be: "A true woman of valor." The phrase, attributed to the description of a wife in Proverbs 31:10-31, describes what perhaps is an idealized lifemate. Susan is and has always been *that* woman of valor.

Hope escapes again. It abandons me on the steps of the temple bema. The future is preordained. I will stand in the ballroom holding Susan in my arms as we waltz to the song of our hearts while she dissolves into a spirit that slips into eternity. With God's grace, I will have the gift of holding her at that moment.

We leave the temple, holding hands, and my soul aches and my eyes tear. I am still thinking about the intersection of their lives—Joan and Susan—that seems to mean only one thing. Susan will be next. For me, Susan has been diagnosed with terminal cancer yet again.

Susan looks up to me and seems to understand. She is silent.

After Joan's death, I again crave normality. I go back to work. Susan is ready for what is next in her life. With the air gone out of the "Elder Affairs" business she and a friend started before the diagnosis, Susan begins to look for a job in the growing independent and assisted living market. It does not take long for the most extensive Jewish senior living facility in nearby Maryland to hire Susan. In theory, the ideal position, except the personalities, or better said, personal work styles, are not a good fit. Susan's style and that of her boss do not mesh. Susan takes her time. She is deliberate, learns routines and methods, and then doggedly pursues them to great success. On the other hand, her boss is an idea-a-minute person, a mover, and a shaker with no patience.

I am on the West Coast when Susan gets fired. She calls to tell me, crying at times, her calm, collected persona shattered. My heart breaks.

"I hate it. I was hoping we could work it out. I walked into my office on Monday, and security comes in to tell me I have been terminated and escorts me out of the building. Why the hell didn't they do it Friday? And why didn't Ellen [her boss] have the guts to talk to me herself? It was humiliating."

Susan has never been fired from anything. The experience hurts her to her core. She never cried like this during any part of her cancer diagnosis or treatment, and I am not there to hold her.

I find little comfort in a phone call. Words evaporate into the wires. As I hear Susan's hurt, I am kicking myself for not being there. "Hold on, Susan, let me get on a plane tonight. I will be home tomorrow."

"No, no. I'm okay. It just hurts."

By the time I get back home later that week, Susan already has drafted a resume for me to look at and lined up job interviews. In classic Susan style, she doesn't obsess about the past; she puts it away somewhere and looks forward. She is determined to find a new position.

In just under six weeks, she gets it done. I am impressed. Once again, in the face of adversity, Susan bears down and moves on. We have such contrasting approaches to life's challenges. I am not the "just move on" kind of guy. I hardly ever take anything in stride. My mind constantly races through alternative courses of action. My what-if-this and what-if-that style has never seemed problematic. To me, it's creative and the right way to live and be prepared. Others see me as a fretter, perhaps even a procrastinator.

This time, Susan, who is definitely not the worrywart, finds her perfect work match. Cedars of Reston is part of a Virginia-based, family-owned-and-run company that operates assisted living facilities in Virginia and Maryland. They hire Susan as director of marketing and admissions. They recognize and respect all her strengths— determination, focus, and intentional pace—that will help her build a strong reputation in the field and build unique solid relationships with the residents.

As Susan thrives in this, her seventh year following the end of treatment, my terror once again slowly fades into the background.

CHAPTER 18

Lynn, My Spiritual Guide

I enter a new phase of this journey. I slowly develop a sense of pride in my role as husband to Susan. It is a conceit that I had been the perfect mate who did everything "just right." I decide that I'm strong. *You made it through the ordeal, and you supported your wife just right.* A new story that I now tell myself. In reality, I was terrified. I assumed the worst and had supernatural visions about ballrooms and orchestras. I buried this existential fear so deep that it has dug its way into my being over the last seven years. I don't realize it is still there, yet it remains, a defect of sorts, a bug in my programming, an existential tectonic scraping or tension as if foreshadowing an earthquake.

By all outward appearances, I am a successful and happy man. My son calls me a "minor celebrity." I am often on television, including an appearance on "The Oprah Winfrey Show." The telecommunication world views me as a leader in the policy field. Clients are happy. Financially, I am doing better than I imagined possible. I can retire.

In reality, amid Joan's death and Susan getting fired, my turmoil and sense of impending doom explode. The earth begins to tremble under me. The clarity of the future still tears at my soul, the scraping more profound and more painful than ever. Something is wrong, broken, or perhaps, only "unfixed."

I wrestle every day with the meaning and purpose of life. I sense that the news of her cancer's return is only a stomachache or headache or backache away. I am distracted from everything else in life and instead focus on what life and love mean. My business and financial success seem meaningless compared to having Susan in my life. I know I am having a crisis, but I don't know how to describe it. The two words that come to mind are spiritual and emotional.

I need to make a change, but I don't know how. Nothing makes sense to me anymore. I am confused and can't manage to connect the dots and relate my anxiety to a core cause—the fear of losing Susan. Those moments of the past, those times of supernatural engagements, also haunt me. The experience with my mother as she took her last breath, once tucked away in irretrievable memory—if there is such a place—seems to stretch and yawn, awakening. The previously grand ballroom no longer appears elegant and beautiful.

I never dare speak of these fears to others. I still have not mentioned them to even Susan in all these years. Unease sits and grows within me. I seek answers on how to live a productive inner life while in a state of constant anticipation of the loss of Susan, the other half of my whole.

Answers come in stages, ever so slowly, through experiential engagements and, sometimes, happenstance. In retrospect, I understand them as necessary steps to reconciliation. Perhaps this is how the universe, or maybe God, speaks to people. It might be that people enter our lives for a reason, like Joan and Stan. And now it is Lynn's turn.

Lynn enters my life at this time when I need her the most. Maybe God, the Divine, brings her into my life to help me out of the existential hole I have dug for myself. This place of spiritual disorder. Of course, I don't realize that at first.

In the spring of 2002, Lynn attends a meeting in Oakland, California, of the World Institute on Disability (WID), on whose board I sit. She will be introduced to the board and then voted on as a member. Lynn and I immediately connect. Though we are both married, our interaction feels a bit like flirting at first. Yet Lynn, who is significantly younger, is about to become a spiritual guide for my recovery from my "PTSD"—post-traumatic spiritual disorder.

As the board meeting comes to a close that day, Lynn takes the initiative. "Let's have lunch, Sam. Come with me. This way."

Wow, I muse. *Lynn's first board meeting, and she already knows where to have lunch. I have been on the board for five years now, and I still don't have any idea of places to eat around here.*

We head out the front door while others schmooze, turn right, and just round the corner is a Vietnamese Restaurant. Lynn has Parkinson's disease (PD) and moves slowly, though with great intention. I have never met someone with Parkinson's before and know little about it. At lunch, we tell our stories. Lynn's speech is slightly impaired, another aspect of her Parkinson's disease. She can sometimes be hard to understand, so I must be attentive. I am entranced.

I find out that Lynn is forty-two, married, and has a ten-year-old daughter. She was diagnosed at age thirty with PD. I interrupt to tell her about Susan and her breast cancer and how deeply I worry about it coming back. Lynn's response is a corrective.

"Listen, Sam, don't feel sorry for yourself. It sounds like Susan has it right. Look at me." Lynn slowly raises both arms out wide. "I am not poor Lynn Fielder, who sadly has PD. I am Lynn with PD. My Parkinson's and I are a whole. We—PD & me—are how we are supposed to be in this world. I am PD Lynn. What I do and how I function is what I'm supposed to be. I will not spend my life feeling sorry for myself and focusing on what I can't do. I focus on what I can do as I am! I will be the best Lynn Fielder ever, no matter what that means in the future."

I am in awe of this extraordinary woman. Lynn is exceptional. The conversation is authentic and oddly intimate, especially for two people who have just met and are now sitting in the middle of this Vietnamese restaurant in downtown Oakland. Enfolded in a personal moment, I see and hear only Lynn.

"So, Sam, Susan isn't poor Susan with breast cancer. You're not poor Sam, whose wife has breast cancer. You are Sam and Susan Simon, who live a life with breast cancer. That is who you are and who you will always be from now on. Now, what are you going to do with that life?"

Deeply affected, I sit and stare in silence. At the moment, I am again in a liminal space, but someplace I don't recognize. It's not the ballroom, and it is for sure not a Vietnamese restaurant in downtown Oakland. I am once again out-of-body, experiencing the world from an entirely different point of view.

Lynn has already made clear by her presence that she is special. She has something to teach me. Not unlike those crazy chance meetings with Joan and Stan, something about this moment seems unusual. We seem to be together for a purpose.

Lynn proceeds to tell me about a book called *The Purpose of Your Life: Finding Your Place In The World Using Synchronicity, Intuition, and Uncommon Sense* by Carol Adrienne. She tells me about Carol's philosophy of following your joy. Carol urges people to listen to how they feel, where they like to be, and what they want to do, and then take steps to change their lives and just do it.

I'm skeptical. The philosophy, as articulated by Lynn, is a little bit out of my comfort zone. I am also curious. I've had my own extraordinary experiences now, but this differs from my spiritual experiences. The ideas sound a bit like what I consider woo-woo or California happy. Perhaps Lynn senses this skepticism.

"Let's go meet Carol," she blurts out. "She's a friend, and she doesn't live that far away."

I am impressed! Lynn's sparkle and energy glow, just as they have throughout this conversation. "Why sure," I say. "When I'm next in town."

"No, right now. Here let me call Carol; she lives only a few miles away. You drive."

Boom, we are off to visit Carol Adrienne, a gracious woman who gladly signs her book after I buy a copy from her. Then we all—Lynn, me, Carol, and Carol's husband—share a glass of wine. I don't think I've ever done anything like this before, running off to have wine and cheese with a well-known author at their home and getting a signed book. Not unusual for Lynn, who once invited herself to lunch with Andy Grove, then President of Intel.

I learn this evening Carol is also a spiritual coach, a numerologist, a Tarot card and palm reader. She likes to meet with people to help guide them into what "should be" their future. I'm bemused and skeptical and figuratively (if not actually) roll my eyes. Her book, though, is mainstream and well-reviewed. It uses case studies to point out that anyone can find purpose or meaning by paying attention to what they naturally like or love to do and then finding the courage to create a life around those things.

The entire experience of being in this alternative environment feels a little cultish, or at least weird. I wonder if I am walking into a place I shouldn't. Lynn enthusiastically encourages me to have Carol read my palm. "Do it, Sam. Don't worry. It will be fine."

Lynn is emphatic, and Carol is more than happy to accommodate. So, we get out my calendar and make an appointment for the next time I am in Oakland. Despite my natural skepticism, I am receptive to it all: synchronicity, Tarot card, and palm readings. Most people who know me would never imagine, I suspect, that I would be open in any way to palm-reading stuff. Heck, I wear a coat and tie to everything. It took a staff rebellion of sorts to convince me to allow Casual Fridays at our office, and I would not dress down myself. Of course, only I know about my out-of-body experiences. Only I know I have seen things I am not supposed to be able to see. Only I experience an ethereal ballroom in a different plane of the universe. So yes, I do believe in a divine connection and supernatural—unexplainable—phenomena.

I quickly learn that Carol pays attention to "coincidences" in life. "Listen to yourself and your joys," she advises. "Follow them." She recommends that I read *Synchronicity: The Inner Path of Leadership*.

Here I am with this woman, a palm reader for goodness sakes, and she suggests a book written by Joseph

Jaworski, the son of Watergate prosecutor Leon Jaworski. I interviewed at Leon Jaworski's law firm for a job while at UT law school in 1969. I can still remember the elegant private luncheon they hosted just to impress me that day. Now I'm reading this book by his son. Yes, I pay attention, and I devour the book.

Joseph Jaworski, it turns out, has a following, generally referred to as groupies. I soon become one of them. In *Synchronicity*, his seminal book though not his only one, Jaworski articulates a belief that all humans are connected by an invisible force with each other and objects. He tells of his search for purpose, describing his encounter with an ermine in the Alps as proof that everything is connected.

The book echoes Carol's theory that there are no accidents, that everything has a purpose, and we just need to listen and learn. Synchronicity is more than coincidence. It's like coincidence with meaning, purpose, and destiny.

Jaworski's description of destiny and coincidence typically cites Martin Buber's *I and Thou,* a book and author I should have known. One might expect that a committed Jewish man like me—former president of his temple—would be familiar with Martin Buber, a leading modern Jewish philosopher. Except I am not, and I am intrigued.

The book's impact on me is fundamental, as significant as Dr. Goldstein's "it's beautiful" moment. Maybe the most meaningful insights come when least expected.

Martin Buber is a philosopher and a theologian most famously known for the idea of a duality of human existence: humans as physical, tangible things or "its," and divine entities or "Thou" beings.

Of course, Susan is my wife in the "it"—or physical world—5'2", bright white hair, and two silicone implants. And she is also a divine presence. A soul. A "Thou."

Buber and Jaworski imagine relationships when two individuals transform to experience each other as divine beings, a manifestation of the breath that God breathed into Adam, which created all life. Indeed, one person can experience another person as a common spiritual manifestation.

As I read the book, it dawns on me that Susan and my relationship has nothing to do with our physicality, the "it" element of being. Buber's articulation of this theory of God's presence, the "Thou" of the other or divine essence experienced between two people, solves a problem for me. It explains how we—Susan and I—can be part of each other. I understand now that Susan and I share that same divine essence. God may well create us as unique beings, but love transforms us, and through that transformation, we exchange sparks of our being with the other. We become a singularity, a Thou. Even though each of us is also an "it," a physically separate man and woman—we are also "us"—a single spiritual being.

I begin to connect my supernatural experiences—the one with my mother that night in George Washington

Hospital and my moments in the ballroom. I now have a framework to understand what has happened and a framework to understand or experience the future.

All this transformation and insight traces back to one person: Lynn Fielder, this incredible lady who turns me on. No, not sexually, though she is attractive. She turns me—the spiritual me, the crazy Sam—on.

As it turns out, a lot is happening in the Bay Area for me, which prompts me to spend an increasing amount of time there. Much of the travel is related to Issue Dynamics. Two of our competitors are in the Bay Area, and I hope to interest one of them in buying Issue Dynamics, or at least my technology business. As it turns out, I end up buying a piece of one firm, bundling it with my company, and selling the package to the other.

In truth, though, the travel is also motivated by wanting to spend more magical time with Lynn. Being with her allows me to stay firmly situated in the everyday world of work, and the parallel world of woo-woo or paranormal, as I search to make normal my time spent in the ballroom.

Susan, in the meantime, continues her road to full strength and energy. She is engaged fully in her new work at Cedars of Reston, which is going very well, and, most importantly, is gaining strength and spirit.

How strange. Susan thrives in her life. I struggle. I search for meaning and purpose in the face of my sense of her inevitable loss. Wanting her to work less and spend more time with me, I push her to travel with me to California. I don't like being away from her this often, especially since stuff seems to happen to her while I'm on the road. She was fired from her first job while I was on the road. Then there was the time when she was in a car accident while I was on the road. I don't want to get a call that she is in the hospital or worse. I also want her to meet Lynn.

Even though business requires less of my presence in Oakland, I still travel as part of my position on the World Institute on Disability board, which allows me to stay close to my captivating new friend. Over this time, Lynn's physical presence changes significantly. She now walks more slowly and with incredible difficulty. I find it harder to understand her words. Her struggles with life's little things contribute to her frustration with WID. She complains that the World Institute on Disability agenda serves only people whose disabilities are permanent and don't change. She, on the other hand, has a progressive disease; her symptoms are getting worse.

"Parkinson's doesn't get better," she reminds me. Then, she shares a short story she has written about her journey. It ends with the following line:

As bad as today seems, I am grateful because I know that things will be worse next year, and I will be looking back to today with envy.

On my next trip to California, Lynn, who lives in Palo Alto, wants to know where I will be staying so she can make a reservation. She wants to stay where I can help her get to the WID Board meeting and back afterward. Kurt, her husband, will drive her to San Francisco for the meeting and pick her up the following morning.

After the Friday-night board meeting, Lynn and I have dinner together back at the San Francisco hotel. Then she insists we visit Grace Church on Nob Hill and walk the labyrinth set up by the church on the front terrace. We arrive by taxi, near midnight. The late-night sky is clear, the temperature a San Francisco warm, and the stars visible. I am in awe of what I already know will be a beautiful and spiritual moment, but I'm also uncomfortable at the same time. On Shabbat evening, a Jewish married man engages in what feels like a pagan ritual with another woman.

Lynn moves slowly. Having gone first, I end up in the center as she is still near the start. She stands as straight as her body will permit. Her mind seems to search for what to do to propel herself forward. She hesitantly steps forward, then swirls backward, then another full swirl around facing forward again. Her arms fly up as if a flamingo dancer—or maybe just flailing—as she takes a small step and moves ahead inches at a time.

I look back at Lynn, who is absorbed in her movements, propelling herself along these twisted, small paths. A peace settles through me. Awash with calmness as if a spiritual rain soaks my soul, I realize this is a perfect

Shabbat. Peace. God is in this place at this moment. I hope Lynn is going to find this same serenity. Maybe this is what this ancient labyrinth ritual is all about—a way to find peace for the soul. Something I will come to understand as love.

Midnight now. Two souls stand together and seemingly struggle with the same questions. In some mysterious way, I wonder if maybe Lynn and I are also meant to be. Standing together at the center of a labyrinth just outside Grace Church here on San Francisco's Nob Hill, it feels like there must be a purpose to the moment and this relationship.

By the time we get back to the hotel, Lynn struggles to move and is slurring her speech. I help her into her hotel room, concerned and confused and very attracted to Lynn in her vulnerability. Should I be here? Is this feeling I have now a betrayal of Susan? Or am I blessed in some way to experience this emotion with more than one person?

The situation is awkward, I think. Can Lynn get herself ready for bed?

She tries to reassure me with her slurred words, "I juhs, juhuhss, just nee, nee, need my meheds, Saa, Sam," she explains. "I shouuuuuld have ta, ta, taken them to be, be, before weeee le, le, left." Her movements are even less reassuring as she leans forward to grab onto something that allows her to slide into the hotel room.

Lynn removes her shoes and enters the bathroom to find her medicine. I peek in after a few minutes to be sure she is okay. My face pops into the bathroom mirror, prompting Lynn to slide the bathroom door closed. A few minutes later, she comes out, grabs my hand, and walks me to the hotel room window. As we stand together looking out at the San Francisco Bay skyline, I experience Lynn not as an "it" but as another soul. I understand this as another Buber's "Thou" moment. I am in awe. Lynn steps back to thank me and send me on my way. She doesn't walk me to the door. Instead, she dismisses me as she sits down on the bed, begins to take off her socks.

Back in my hotel room, I want to share the moment with Susan. I pick up the phone, start to dial, and realize the time. It is 4 a.m. in McLean, Virginia. I'd better wait until morning.

Susan comes with me to Oakland for the next WID board event. The trip will provide us with a short vacation and allow Susan to meet Lynn. When Lynn, Susan, and I finally get together, the two of them are like sisters. Susan proudly wears the necklace, crafted by Lynn, that I gave Susan for our fortieth wedding anniversary. Susan understands my attraction to Lynn, who has become a spiritual guide to discovering the interconnectedness of all beings and all things.

Not surprisingly, in this discovery process, I find a sense of oneness with Lynn, and intimacy and inevitability that seem like some mystic source has created them. Perhaps every human being's divine essence is vaster than we can know and is available to be shared infinitely with many others. The test or challenge, the mystery, is why and how that connection awakens between any two people.

Lynn's gifts of insight and connection have never left me, and Lynn continues to be a friend, although her journey has left her in an even more impaired state. At the time, my encounters with Lynn and Carol and my explorations of spiritual worlds bound me more deeply into Susan. I now understand, feel, or perhaps just sense that love and divinity are synonyms and have a concrete expression in relationships. So, now, even in our forty-first year of marriage, Susan and I can experience deeper intimacy in our relationship. I also begin to understand more concretely the ballroom as a manifestation of our intimate and infinite connection. My disappearance for endless moments into liminal space and time of a transitional ballroom to hold Susan as she leaves is also a "Thou" moment, an instant of near oneness with the divine.

As much as I appreciate these insights, my life now and for the foreseeable future is divided between newfound intimate moments with Susan and moments of unimaginable fear and confusion. I am dizzy and torn by these radical shifts between newfound moments of physical and emotional intimacy with Susan and reminders of the precipice of an end. In bed, holding Susan, I now inhale her breath, and it becomes our breath. Then as my hands touch her face and slide down her neck to her chest, suddenly I am awake to cancer. The fingers slide from smooth skin onto the silicone implants' rough texture tightly contained in taut skin. I press gently, then am verbally slapped by Susan's terse, "Sam, I don't feel anything. That area is dead to me. Leave them alone." Intimacy, breath, and cancer fill the spaces of my life. Adjust, adapt, and move on.

Moving on can make life seem routine at times. Maybe this is normal. Perhaps the orchestra is gone, never to return. Maybe my spiritual disorder is finally over.

The passage of time tricks the mind into doubting the past. Perhaps this is just how the mind works, how it resolves or makes tolerable spiritual disorder. As time passes, I begin to doubt my own experience and the truth of the ballroom.

CHAPTER 19

Gaining Clarity

*M*y doubting stops on January 10th, 2010, a few months shy of the ten-year mark of coming home to Susan's: "Just one more thing, Sam."

The telephone rings on January 3rd, a week before that day. Susan and I are just back from spending a great New Year's weekend at LodgeBend with our children and grandchildren in Virginia's Northern Neck. LodgeBend is the name we have given our second home, located two and a one-half hours from our home in McLean. The driveway to the house sits at a bend in the road that parallels Lodge Creek, a small body of water that flows into the Potomac, not far from the Chesapeake Bay.

I hear Rabbi Laszlo Berkowits's anxious voice on the phone. "Sam, you need to come. You're up!"

Rabbi Berkowits is now the rabbi emeritus of Temple Rodef Shalom, the Reform Jewish temple Susan and I joined in 1973, and where we have both been president of the congregation. He and I have become close friends.

"What are you talking about?"

"Dick is in the ICU. He fell. It's serious. You're his power of attorney. You need to come. It might be the end."

Boom. All that time of seeming normality vanishes in an instant, and I am back in the middle of a spiritual vortex.

"Dick" is Rabbi Richard Sternberger, a friend of thirty-plus years, who served as the adjunct rabbi to our temple for most of that time. A righteous man and an icon of the civil rights movement in the United States, he has been a clarion voice for social justice in the Jewish reform community to the world. We became close friends, driven by our mutual love for dogs and our shared passion for social justice. "We" includes Susan, Marcus, Rachael, our dogs Lucky and Maddie, and his giant sheepdogs. Over time, Dick had three—Tory, then Falstaff, and then Stuart.

When Dick and I had lunch together on December 31st, 2009, just eleven days prior, he seemed perfectly fine. He was in a righteous rage, insisting that we change his will as his first priority in the new year. I happen to be the executor of his estate, and I have a power of attorney to act on his behalf if ever needed. We agreed to get together early in 2010 to make these changes. We wish each other a wonderful new year and head off from what we could not know would be our last routine interaction with each other.

"Over the weekend, Dick fell and hit his head on a concrete sidewalk," Rabbi Berkowits explains. "He did not lose consciousness. Insisting his injury was minor, Dick refused treatment. The next day, Monday, he collapsed and was rushed to the hospital. He is now critical. You need to come right away! Bring all your papers. The hospital says they need them."

On the afternoon of January 3rd, 2010, I rush to Inova Fairfax hospital, go up to the ICU, walk into a room, and look at my semi-conscious friend. I have been down this road before. I can already picture the end. It is as if I were back in 2000 sitting in a narrow closet-like room staring at a piece of paper that painted the end of Susan.

Today, it is different and yet the same. Even though Dick is not a relative, I must play the next-of-kin role with my friend, teacher, and fellow dog lover. Just as I did with Susan and my mother, except he is no longer conscious. I don't have to hold out small semi-circle pans for him to throw up. He has a catheter, so I don't have to help him to the bathroom. I don't sleep over. Still, I am back in hospital mode, which triggers my memories of getting ready for what I was so sure would be Susan's death.

This journey isn't just about my friend, the righteous Rabbi Richard Sternberger. It is also about Susan. Susan, who also loves Dick Sternberger, is also with me in the hospital each day, navigating the delicate process of end-of-life rituals. And yes, she is more stoic than I am. She keeps me centered and steady.

Over the next eight days, I manage Rabbi Dick Sternberger's end-of-life journey. I have the responsibility to decide if and how his life will end. Do we take extraordinary measures or not? He is now on life support; the oxygen administered through a mask keeps him breathing. Fluids entering his body provide hydration and some nourishment. If we remove them, the doctors tell me he will die. How long should he be kept on life support?

My spiritual disorder explodes. How the hell do I make this decision? I have a bit of a conflict of interest here. I need to be true to my "client's" wishes. After all, he has trusted me as his medical representative, and he has expressed his desires. Yet, I have a deep loving relationship with my friend. I stand this night in his hospital room and recall, indeed relive, that moment in my mother's hospital room as she took her last breath and my vow then never again to withhold extraordinary measures. I decided back then that we should always take every available action to prolong life for every second possible, which, I have since learned, might be an eon in universal time.

I also desperately want Dick to recover.

As I struggle with what to do, I begin to get contradictory advice from medical professionals.

"Give him some time. I have seen people suddenly wake up," I hear from a young neurosurgeon, a young man who had grown up in our temple and knew him as "Uncle Dick."

"It's over," other doctors insist. "He has no hope of recovery. If he survives, he will be in a semi-vegetated state."

How do I make the decision?

"Follow your heart," says Susan.

My heart says, "Don't stop." A thought also burdens me. *Is this just a rehearsal for Susan? If I decide to withhold treatment for Rabbi Sternberger now, how can I deal with Susan when faced with this same decision?*

I am confused. I don't want to do this myself. It takes me a long, agonizing weekend to figure out what action to take. I decide not to make this decision myself. Yes, I have the authority to do so; Dick placed his trust in me when he designated me his medical power of attorney. His ex-wife predeceased him, and he has no children. His other best friend, Rabbi Berkowits—beside himself with guilt and grief for having been with Dick when he fell— now tells me he does not want to be part of this decision.

I realize that others have a deep, loving relationship with this incredible human being, and they deserve a voice in this decision. Their hearts and souls are also aching at this moment. While I have authority, I decide to share the burden and bring a small group of these friends and cousins into the process—individuals who love him and who may also have a strong opinion about, or reaction to, any decision we make.

At 8 p.m. on Thursday, January 7th, 2010, Dick still lies in a shared bay, or suite of sorts, on an urgent care floor, a level of care area between the ICU and the regular-care room. The group of us, eight people who love him, meet outside the room. Together we silently enter the room. He is not conscious, but who knows if he isn't above just watching?

I speak, calling out the name of each person as I do. "Please say now if you agree that the time has come, according to Dick's wishes, to end treatment."

A sacred presence fills the room during an infinite pause, which may only be a second or two. Then each person looks at Dick and me and says aloud so I and perhaps Dick can hear, *yes*. Each of us takes a private moment with him, touching him, saying something, and then leaves the room.

Later that night, Dick is transferred from the shared bay on the hospital's urgent care floor to a private room. We call in hospice care. Susan and I are by his side from morning to evening. On Friday, January 8th, hospice tells us his end is near. If we remove his oxygen, he will stop breathing, they say. We arrange for people who want to come to visit over the weekend. As I leave the room that Friday night, I have the nurse tune the radio to the station that plays opera around the clock. Dick loves opera. It will stay on for the rest of his life.

Monday, January 10th, 2010, I arrive back in his room at 7 a.m.

I am, once again, alone in the room. Hospice walks in around 8 a.m. We turn the radio sound down, but not off. They look at me, and we nod toward each other—no counting down this time. Instead, a nurse simply removes the oxygen mask, and Dick's rhythmic gasps stop. A doctor walks over, places a stethoscope on his chest, then turns to me. "He's gone," she says.

I wait expectantly. What will happen this time? I don't know if I want to see a spinning tuft of white cloud leave him or not. Would it cheapen the experience with my mother? Nothing happens. The room is quiet. A hospice nurse pulls the light blanket over his face.

Once again, I have some calls to make. We all leave the room to the hospital staff for proper cleaning and preparation until the funeral home staff can collect his body.

People begin to arrive. Rabbi Berkowits, Dick's best friend, and Rabbi Schwartzman, now senior rabbi of the temple, are the first to join me. Susan leaves work and rushes over. We all talk, share memories, make plans, and I cry. No, I sob. *What is this?* I don't cry like this in front of people. I look at Susan. And wonder if my crying is for what might have been—or what might yet be—for her, as well as the death of my friend.

The following Saturday, Susan and I arrive as usual for Shabbat morning services at our temple. The once-a-month "alternative" service occurs in a small, intimate space in our temple's downstairs area. We are away from the main sanctuary, which is much larger and typically features several young people celebrating their B'nai Mitzvah. We greet friends as we walk in when the rabbi comes up to me and asks:

"Sam, are you comfortable saying a few words about Dick?"

"Of course," I reply. "Thank you."

I know what I am going to say. I will offer a few sentences from the eulogy I gave at Dick's funeral just a few days earlier.

"We were related by dog."

"He was an icon of Jewish social justice."

"He taught us all that 'the meaning of life is to live a life of meaning.' "

I settle in. Services begin with the beautiful, soft, high-pitched voice of Rabbi Saxe, an ordained rabbi and an invested cantor. He is playing the guitar, a niggun, to bring us all into the room.

Suddenly a sharp pain sears deep inside my head. Every muscle in my body tightens as my mind screams. This is new! Different! It is as if a hammer or an ax has split my brain in half without touching the skull.

I freeze, then grab onto Susan's arm, squeezing so tight that I alarm her. I think I am about to pass out. *Oh my God, I'm having a stroke!*

Then I hear it boldly resonate inside my head— the distinct, unmistakable deep, gravelly, familiar Dick Sternberger voice. "Don't worry, Sam. Everything is going to be okay." Then nothing, just silence. As the service begins, my body relaxes, and my head feels fine. I want to ask what he means, why I need to know or hear these words. What is "everything?" *Is this a dream? A hallucination? Am I just anxious?*

No, I feel perfectly comfortable and confident. I look at Susan, who had whispered, "Is everything okay?" I whisper back, "Yes." I take her hand in mine, and we sit holding hands for the next few minutes.

"As you all know, our beloved Rabbi Dick Sternberger passed away this past week," I hear the rabbi announce. "I've asked his dear friend, Sam Simon, to say a few words about Dick this morning. Please come up, Sam."

I stand up before that small Saturday morning congregation and say all the things I planned, with one slight change: "I know Dick is here in the room with us this morning and that everything is okay."

As the service ends, and the rabbi offers us a few moments for silent reflection. I close my eyes. I can see that giant spinning tuft of a white cloud as it exited my mother over forty years ago as if it were yesterday. I remember her spirit or soul leaving the room and feel validated in my belief that what I saw was real. Hearing Dick's voice this morning has left me reinforced in the knowledge that a significant force in the universe exists, which connects each of us. I feel blessed.

CHAPTER 19

A New Intimacy

The most important gifts in my life come in unexpected ways and often during great pain. This incredible paranormal experience with my beloved rabbi and friend, which has carried me back to the events of 2000 and the memories from 1973 in my mother's room, validate the truths of those experiences. Despite Susan's current health and strength, I immediately interpret this moment as a form of training to prepare myself for the unthinkable and to be with Susan at her last breath.

I am once again at the bottom of the emotional roller-coaster. Are we going to walk into our home after this Saturday morning service and see the voice-mail light on the phone with a call from the oncologist asking Susan to come in again for something? I get it—my fears are irrational. She has not been to the doctor in nearly two years. And that is the nature of the roller-coaster.

I don't tell Susan about any of this. Instead, after we get home this Saturday and have our Shabbat lunch, we have sex. Holding her, kissing her, she fills me up with her breath and her essence. I yearn for it every day.

Life and death. Or is it love and death? I've since read a book where the author makes the bold assertion that the opposite of death is not life; it is love. Love is not an emotion, and life is not a journey. They are both states of being. The journey is the search or experience of those moments, perhaps Martin Buber's "Thou" moments. Maybe this is something else I will come to understand.

The hard reality is that everyday human life and emotions are just barriers to finding something more profound. The challenge is to figure out how to get past the pain and pleasures of commonplace experiences to discover a path from "it" to "Thou" relationships.

I am not a guru nor a spiritual master who transcends the real world to live in some ecstatic state. I am Samuel A. Simon, who seems to be on an extraordinary life journey, privileged to experience what seems like levels of being that others find difficult to find. Someone needs to tell me why. I don't understand. What I do instead is to build on the deeply held terror of anticipated loss as a marker for how much I love Susan. A division between the soul of a being and the tangibility of existence.

Nonetheless, we begin to experience some signs of progress together. In 2010, a decade after Susan's original diagnosis and nine years after her last treatment, Susan is scheduled for her "final appointment." It is a formal, real-world end to Susan's breast cancer journey.

Susan's current oncologist is a woman. She had been in practice with Dr. Blonder during Susan's treatment period and took over the case when Dr. Blonder retired two years earlier.

"Wow, Susan, what a journey you have had! You look great." She knows that Susan, who someone recently described as "buff," exercises every day now. Her biceps are apparent!

"As far as we are concerned, the cancer is gone! Your blood tests are normal. You don't need to come back unless something new comes up. Your primary doctor will keep an eye on things." In other words, Susan's oncologist dismisses her as a cancer patient. Yes, she is always going to be known or tagged as a survivor. Indeed, our next decade will continue to be one Avon Walk after another, with pink ribbons for Susan, designating her as a walking survivor. We are a "Pink Family," it seems, forever.

It takes only a few months for something else to come up, another unexpected and oddly encouraging moment in this cancer journey.

"Sam, my left implant feels funny. It hurts. Can you see anything?"

I look, I squeeze it a little, and I can tell that, yes, something is wrong. It feels like a half-empty bag of liquid, as if some of the silicon has leaked. The left breast is softer and squishier than the right side.

Susan hunts down the cosmetic surgeon who performed the original reconstruction back in 2000. No easy task a decade-plus after the surgery.

The surgeon remembers Susan. "You know, Susan, we mentioned when you opted for the implants that their normal life span is ten years," she reminds her.

Yes! Susan has outlived her breast implants. Maybe we should have a breast-implant replacement celebration dinner. Or a party. Can we have sex?

Susan and I haven't talked about our evolving relationship. We both just seem to be living it. My ecstatic reaction to her implant replacement amuses her, and her response is almost condescending. I sometimes think she can smell my fear underneath the façade of celebration. "Get over it, Sam" is her way of being... not angry, not frustrated or frustrating, just matter-of-fact, just Susan.

We begin to develop affirmation rituals—little things in everyday life that were not present before cancer. Every night before we go to sleep, we kiss each other goodnight. Sometimes just a peck, sometimes more. Each morning, we kiss each other goodbye and say, "I love you." I notice, too, that our daughter has picked up the habit. She ends every phone call with "Love you." Yes, so easy for these routines to become just that—routine, mechanical—but not for Susan, me, nor our daughter.

Susan and I experience our lives together as a second chance, a level of daily joy and gratitude different from BBC, before Susan got sick. Over time, the line between

ABC and BBC—after breast cancer and before breast cancer—grows brighter. The reality of life itself seems more routine every day. Perhaps even mundane. We are just people who get irritated with petty things and each other. We have good days and bad days. Like others, we need our quiet time, our different relationships.

Yet now, every night, we are together. Every morning when we wake up, we are where we are supposed to be. Indeed, maybe this all has happened to strengthen us for even more significant life challenges.

CHAPTER 20

Toward a New Era

*C*hanges in our external worlds mirror this internal evolution of increased intimacy, especially in our work lives. My ongoing struggle with professional purpose culminates in late 2008 when I sell the remaining part of my company to a colleague and friend. At a small celebration in our offices, I stand in our large conference room to thank and congratulate the new owner.

The emotions of different moments in the twenty-two-year history flick through my body. The uncertainty of my start, the energy of new clients, the funny random incidents, the gratitude for when the staff embraced me not so long ago during Susan's cancer, the confusion I have endured throughout Susan's illness, and which I continue to endure.

Yet, in this new era of my soul, I shed no tears and do not mourn a loss for what has been only a moment in time. This moment, which acknowledges the end of the company that has served me so well, is not death, nor is it a massive victory of some sort. Indeed, it is merely a moment in time. My energy and emotions focus on relationships, love, and meaning in life's journey. Perhaps the grinding spiritual disorder has liberated me from caring about business activities, even if it hasn't yet liberated me from work itself.

The crushing deadlines of due diligence and wrapping up a complex sale don't leave me a lot of time to obsess about what's next in life. Fortunately, my new way in the world allows me to trust that the right thing will appear. Right on cue, it does. Shortly after the sale announcement, my friend, Reverend Robert Chase, who lives and works in Cleveland, Ohio, calls me.

"Sorry I couldn't be at the announcement of the sale, Sam," says Bob, with whom I worked for some twenty years. "I just got into town. How about breakfast for old times' sake. I have some important news to share, and I want to do it in person."

We meet the next day at the Mayflower Hotel. My lox-and-bagels obsession is a running joke between Bob and me. He knows I insist on having that for breakfast as part of my diet, and he makes sure to choose a restaurant that satisfies the requirement.

"I'm leaving the UCC (United Church of Christ) and moving to New York to lead a new social justice ministry at the Collegiate Churches of New York," he says.

I learn that the Collegiate Churches of New York— the oldest church in the United States, chartered in

1628—has been comprised of four unique ministries. Norman Vincent Peale was once the minister at Marble Collegiate Church, the largest of the ministries. They recently launched their fifth ministry, a new multi-ethnic, multi-faith initiative called Intersections International. They have hired Bob to lead the work. Their goal for the organization is to work "on the front lines of national and global conflict to bring greater understanding, love, and healing to our world." They have set aside twenty million dollars for a ten-year commitment.

He is not here just to tell me about the project. He wants me to go to New York early next year to participate in a brainstorming session with the small staff and several other "friends of Bob" to envision the project and figure out how to go about changing the world. To be fair, he may not have explicitly used the words *changing the world*, but that is how I interpret this incredible opportunity.

Indeed, during this conversation, I experience a spiritual tickle. *Maybe this is where I belong? What I should be doing?* As soon as I get home, I fill Susan in on the development. It occurs to me that Susan has by now sensed my spiritual disorder. We never talk about it, and that failure has created perhaps a tiny barrier between us. We both know something is going on with me, and we are both afraid to get too near it.

Despite what may just be a subconscious lapse, we seek ways to help each other be happy and strong in life. As always, I shield Susan from my ever-present belief that, despite the evidence, cancer will come back. Susan searches for ways to restore my spirit. So, when she senses new energy in my words and the twinkle of the possibility of being part of something new, she encourages me. "It will be exciting for you, Sam. Don't worry about me. I'm so, so busy at work."

I *am* excited. The opportunity reminds me of my early days with Ralph Nader. A start-up social justice initiative with an incredible platform in New York. Yes, I'm audacious enough to think I might have the opportunity to change the world.

Over the weekend, I write Bob a letter, yes, a letter that I sign and mail, telling him just that—we can change the world, and imagining how together we can make a difference.

Bob is a cautious man. It will take a bit to work things out. "Expect a *yes* by spring." Perfect for me. I need to finalize my exit from the firm and settle into my emeritus role as chairman, a two-year commitment intended to reassure existing clients.

As the spring approaches and my role as a senior fellow with Intersections clearly defined, I begin to struggle with the prospect of being away from Susan for half of every month. I still worry about her health. I always listen for a new and different orchestra to form and for Susan and me to appear in the center of a ballroom, ready to dance the actual dance.

"Sam, I am fully capable of being home alone for ten days a month," she says. My first reaction is to tell her to "just stop it." I realize that I sound like Susan, telling her to stop trying to fix me. She doesn't understand that the big breast cancer bogeyman is just outside the door, about to walk in and swallow her. Inside, I am the knight with the shield keeping that bogeyman away. In reality, I am suffocating her, but I just don't see that, and I don't stop.

"Why don't you quit your job, Susan? We don't need the money! Come spend the time in New York with me." I even suggest that we buy an apartment in New York and split our time between McLean, New York, and our house in the Northern Neck.

To be honest, I find the prospect of having a residence in three separate places a bit alluring. We could do it. I have been reckless before. In 1977, I left the federal government while making a significant income to return to work with Ralph Nader at half that salary and after we bought a new house in McLean, Virginia. Now, all it would take is a little financial finagling—perhaps a refinance of our main home or another mortgage. Maybe we could find friends who would partner with us to buy a New York place that we could share.

In a manic response to good fortune and almost the opposite end of the vertical universe, I soar up from the depths of the bogeyman that will cause Susan's death to the infinite height of the "us" of Susan and me forever. We can do whatever we want together and forever.

Susan doesn't want to go. She is now highly regarded in the eldercare community in Northern Virginia and is the director of marketing and admissions at Cedars of Reston. She often leads training at other properties owned by the Cedars' owners. Her work gives her new meaning and energy. Why would she want to give that up? Of course, I see only the cancer-Susan, and I just want to be with her.

Eventually, Susan's strong encouragement and determined persistence in urging me to follow my heart win the day. The first few months, we just talk on the phone every night. Every call ends with "I love you" from her and a "ditto" from me, a nod to the movie *Ghost*, our favorite. The phone call reassures me that she is, for the moment, okay. With the advent of the iPhone, we start to FaceTime each night. The "I love you" now is followed by "ditto" and a virtual kiss. Alone in an apartment in New York, I turn off the lights and play "Unchained Melody" on my iPhone and let it take me to sleep.

New York is perfect medicine for my spiritual disorder. The most unexpected joy comes from the role of being just one member of a team with no responsibility for revenue nor management of people. I love, I mean *love*, not being the boss. From 1978 to 2009, for about thirty-one years, I was not just the boss. I was literally on the line financially for the entire firm. Now I am merely one of the people working at Intersections, an employee. The loss of responsibility oddly energizes me. I am thrilled!

As the proverbial icing on the cake in New York, the world capital of theater, I find a way to pursue my passion for improv and acting. I discovered improv in my mid-fifties through a fellow actor one summer. She introduced me to a small group of actors connected to a New York theater group called Artistic New Directions, or AND.

Starting in the summer of 2002, I attend AND retreats in the Catskills, near Woodstock, New York. The retreat features an intensive improv workshop taught by a world-class faculty. At first, I'm a beginner, and I struggle, really struggle as I compare myself to many twenty-something aspiring actors from New York City. Each year as I leave the retreat, driving home by myself down windy rural New York roads, my body feels like I have been bared naked as a pretender. I swear never to return. I want to jump into an ice-covered pond to stop the searing soul pain of perceived failure. Yet the improv experience awakens something very deep inside of me. So, in the end, I return year after year to suffer. I now wonder if the feeling is about the real me at that time in my life.

Improv is about letting go of the outside world to be fully present at the moment, of authentic relationships with the other actors on stage with you. It is akin to the Martin Buber challenge of seeing the divine, as opposed to the other's 'it.' When on stage, my job is to accept all information given and add to it. To experience and honor my fellow actors and help them be their best self on stage at that exact moment. Improv is living life authentically in every scene on stage, which requires me to open up to the fire that still burns deep inside me—the certainty of losing Susan. Maybe that is what starts to happen each year as I drive away from the Full Moon Resort feeling like I am on fire, swearing never to return or subject myself to what now feels so painful.

By 2008, my improviser skills have grown, and the moments on stage energize me instead of exposing me. Now that I am an every-other-week resident of New York City, I can spend time at AND's Tuesday and Wednesday night classes. I also manage to attend as many of their events as possible, including classes and workshops with various teachers, to the point where I become a regular member of the Artistic New Directions team in Washington and New York. Who could have imagined? I'm changing the world and performing on stage in New York and Washington as an improviser!

CHAPTER 22

Letting Go and Acting Up

*M*y life soon becomes schizophrenic. I live in two worlds. At one moment, I can be on stage in New York or hosting a conference on ethical leadership at the Yale Club. And the next instant, I exit into the grand ball-room, holding Susan in my arms for our final waltz, called there by a casual comment from Susan. The "I'm tired" during our nightly check-in call. Or, at home, complaints of a headache. Despite the passage of time, I am just barely holding on. I still listen. I still know the end is inevitable. Life is full of reminders.

Just a month into this new life, I get a telephone call. Tom, a close friend from the Ralph Nader days, wants me to know that our former colleague, Gary, has died. His family will host a memorial service at a church in Northern Virginia, not far from where Susan and I live.

Gary, a one-of-a-kind type of guy, was already working for Ralph Nader when Tom and I started back in 1970.

Mysterious in his ways, secretive in his actions, and sometimes just plain weird, he was a behind-the-scenes worker in all of Ralph's early auto safety campaigns, including those that resulted in anti-rollover designs and mandatory seat belts. Ironically, Gary died when a jeep he was driving, without a seat belt, rolled over.

A few of us from the 1970 era who worked with Gary attend the memorial service. When I step through the church's doors for the memorial service, a sense of calm, quiet, and beauty fully engrosses me. I stop and take a breath. As I absorb late morning, summer light shines through beautiful stained-glass windows, and the soft sound of the organ music fills the room. People chat quietly. I see a seat open next to Tom, slide in, and dissolve into the moment.

Silly me! What makes me think I can confront death without thinking about Susan, without that old traumatic energy that hovers inside bursting into the bright present. Once again, I am pretending that the spiritual disorder had passed. *Would these people have come if it had been Susan's funeral nearly ten years ago?* I wonder. Then, feeling self-indulgent, I try to shake myself back into the present.

After reading from Christian scripture, the minister welcomes us and introduces Sally, Gary's widow. "I know it sounds odd, but there is one good thing about Gary's death," she says during her eulogy. "I asked him once to tell me his greatest fear. His answer, 'You predeceasing me.' Well, Gary, lucky you, you did not have to live your worst nightmare."

I forget to breathe as I sit still and motionless. In that instant, I realize that I am Gary. I have never heard those words spoken out loud before. My worst fear. Gary's worst fear. Love's worst fear. I have walked up to the precipice. Indeed, I live there.

A piece of my puzzle falls into place. How weird. Nearly a decade into this journey with Susan, I sit here, having walked in with the conceit that I had left behind my spiritual disorder. Of course not. The ache, the confusion, is still there, deep down inside, suddenly yanked up to the top by a simple sentence.

I experience validation, as well. I am not alone. I want to scream, "Gary, you lucky bastard, you didn't have to live your worst fear. You died first. You didn't even have to face the possibility." I wonder if Sally can be so composed and comfortable speaking to this room because she didn't have to be with her husband for months as he slowly died. She didn't have to anticipate it. Instead, the phone rang, and she knew Gary was gone. It was over. I begin to feel a slight resentment that Sally can be so smug, so confident in what she is saying about Gary and herself. She talks about his death so nonchalantly. She even says she is happy that Gary was doing something he loved in his final moments, as the Jeep rolled over on him. I could not imagine anything giving me peace should Susan predecease me. Period.

Yes, Susan did not die. This fact should be my ultimate joy. Except for me, her illness is not over. I continue to anticipate the realization of that worst fear, along with the infinite intimacy of the end—that unimaginable, inevitable moment with Susan. I live it just as a soldier relives the moment of the roadside bomb that went off and killed his buddy. Unpredictably, triggered by things that I don't see coming, the explosion propels me into the ballroom, holding Susan, waltzing to the end. I still know what is going to happen.

I am jealous of Gary and Sally—Gary for predeceasing Sally, and Sally for her calm and loving ability to tell this story.

Not long after Gary's funeral, I head to my next Artistic New Directions improv retreat, once again at the Full Moon Resort near Woodstock, New York. This year, improvisational master teacher Gary Austin has brought a student from California. Gary has been working with Craig Nelson to develop a performance based on a recent experience in Craig's life. That's an improv technique: Tell a story, write it down, and then perform it.

Craig reads from his script. He has written a true story about when, as a volunteer mountain rescuer, he is called to help retrieve the body of a young boy lost in California's mountains. Craig finds the body and carries it back to the parents. He describes seeing the family out in the front yard, along with crowds of neighbors standing around on a California evening just before sunset. Craig's script includes his thoughts during the ride to the boy's home with the dead boy in his lap. Holding the body is a way for him to meld himself into what had been this child's spirit, so when he hands him to the parents, he does so with empathy and shared tragedy. He describes sensing the moment as occurring in slow motion: slowly stepping out of the car and walking across a lawn while feeling at the same time above the scene.

I am nauseous as I absorb the story. The fuse, lit just a few weeks ago at Gary's funeral, burns hot inside of me. My spiritual disorder is screaming. I know Craig's experience differs from mine, but his language regarding the spiritual impact resonates deeply. I have lived that moment in my soul. The sense of fear and grace he articulates, the pain he can anticipate each time his phone rings with the call to head for the retrieval, and then the dignity of how he returns the body to the parents spark an image. Perhaps this is the end of my fuse—the end, my end, as I hold the weight of Susan's lifeless body once the orchestra stops playing and her essences escape. Of course, how have I missed that most tragic moment that will occur in the ballroom? This "aha" comes nearly a decade later at the retreat.

During this incredibly emotional moment, I wonder if I, too, might have a story to tell. As Craig ends his reading, the room is silent. As we collectively seem to be holding our breath, a loud noise in my head shouts: "Tell your story. Tell the damned story." I wonder if I can. Even thinking about it scares me.

Bits and pieces of my story begin to pop into my head during acting classes as I take my turn. The memory of moments so long ago now begins to bubble to the surface and flood back into my throat. The moments, the smells, the words are here, alive, inside of me.

I start to give expression to it all—the day Susan's mother dies, the extraordinary events of my mother's death, the diagnosis, the ever more challenging news related to her condition.

As I tell these pieces over time in different classes, my classmates and teachers respond. "More, more. Give us more!" Surprised and motivated, I write, write, and write, and I give them more.

I begin to sense the value for me of being able to tell my story. I write and rewrite myself. I show drafts to various theater friends and coaches. I hear that what I wrote is too long, too short, too confusing. Occasionally I hear, "Why don't you write about something more fun and joyful?"

Finally, my acting teacher tells me I need a dramaturg, a person who goes over the script, asks questions, and guides the writer to a dramatic presentation of the story. It turns out that one of my classmates in New York is also a dramaturg. Gabrielle Maisels has already heard bits and pieces and is excited to help.

Gabrielle and I meet every two weeks. "Sam, you are ready to start sharing this with others," she says after three short months. "The next step is to begin reading and getting feedback."

On that day in New York, at the Intersection's offices, as I read what I have written to a small group of friends and fellow actors, I begin to lose confidence. I feel like a fraud, and maybe everyone is just playing with me.

In the end, I receive a standing ovation from this small group. I'm astonished. Gabrielle is *k'velling*—the Jewish phrase for someone proud of their work. Megan says how important it is to hear a man's voice talk about breast cancer. Fred pulls me over to the side to tell me about his cancer experience. This experience will become the norm. Women speak out loud about the show, and men come up for private sidebars to talk about their reactions.

I spend many days that summer reading what I have written to small New York audiences. Lots of different groups. I go to one more improv retreat and read the draft to a group of my theater friends, those of us who have "played" together every summer for about eight years. Their love and energy for this story humble me. One of the young students from California announces to all the "campers" at the end-of-retreat goodbye circle that hearing this reading was the most meaningful retreat event. More than that, it was the most critical event in her entire life!

It may also be among the most critical moments in my own life. It is the moment I notice a change in me. The sense of fear of that fuse burning toward an emotional implosion begins to diminish. My soul comes alive as I experience the audience respond to the play. Love. The empathy of "thank you; it's exactly how I felt." Responses. The quiet asides of appreciation. I internalize them all. It feels imperative to keep the work going. The gift to me, perhaps the most significant gift of all, is that I begin to experience, to know, that I am not alone. So many others share this journey, struggle as I struggle, and I find deep comfort in this understanding.

CHAPTER 23

Telling Susan

I have a problem. Susan and I still live on different planes of the universe, with her fully immersed in her growing success at work and me in the middle of perhaps the most important discovery of my life—writing and performing the play that is resolving my spiritual disorder. Susan knows I am involved in improv and writing. While in New York, I tell her about working on a one-person show, but I don't reveal any details other than that the show is about something I have been working on in class. "A story." I have yet to share what I was feeling at the time of her illness. I don't know how to tell her about the play.

Susan is aware of a change in me. She senses it and occasionally mentions how happy I seem with my improv work in New York and my work with Intersections and our social justice initiatives. I'm sure she's relieved that I have stopped begging her to quit her job and be in New York with me.

Two events combine to create a crisis of revelation. First, friends invite me to read the play in their apartment to a small audience on the Tuesday after Labor Day, 2012. Second, our friends from Canada, Ken and his wife Ginny, will be in New York for the Labor Day weekend.

Susan can come to New York to enjoy the weekend and be with Ken and Ginny. She needs to get back home Monday so she can be at work early Tuesday. In theory, this will let me continue sidestepping the inevitable moment of truth since she will miss the play. The problem with my idea is that Ken and Ginny will stay over and attend the reading. They are excited about it. They have also experienced a devastating loss. About a decade earlier, during a school trip to Costa Rica, they lost their son, Morgan, when he was just sixteen years old. So, they have danced "the actual dance."

The jig is up, of course. Susan needs to know what the hell is going on. *The Actual Dance*, my then-working title for the play, doesn't reveal anything to her, but she will find out. What should I do?

No, I am not going to just sit in our living room and read it to her. I have been writing for almost two years without ever telling her the play is about her death from breast cancer. Do I think she will get angry? Do I think she will just believe it is too personal? Is she going to demand that I stop?

Maybe the reason behind my avoidance is that I still believe the story is not over. I am afraid Susan will hear that I still think she is going to die. I don't want her to hear me say that I know in my soul the cancer is just asleep inside her, and it will one day wake up. And yet, she is going to have to know.

I can't avoid the moment any longer. I've got to figure something out. I decide to let Susan read the script that Saturday as we take the train to New York. Yes, on the train to New York. I admit it is unfair. I think doing it this way may limit her options and box her in. I know Susan. Her default is to be private. She has no interest in the world hearing about her breast cancer or my reactions.

We are on the Acela (the fast train from DC to New York), leaving Baltimore. The next stop is not for about an hour. Susan is reading the newspaper.

"Susan, here's the play I have been writing. I need you to read it." I hand her a pink, plastic three-ring flexible binder. Susan takes it and begins to read. She starts to cry, and then reads more and cries, and reads, and then sobs. No explanation, no anger. She just keeps reading. Uncomfortable and uncertain about what her reaction means, I look around the train car and notice that a few people seem to be glancing over.

When Susan finishes the script, she slowly lays it on her lap and turns to me. "I am so sorry, Sam." She struggles to talk through her tears. She hugs me and kisses me—and people's glances turn to stares. "I didn't know you were going through this. I had no idea."

I am relieved and surprised. It had not occurred to me that there was yet another secret in this drama. My effort to support Susan by mirroring her determination was successful. She did not see that desperate fear inside of me for all these years. I hid it at the time and continued to do so for eleven years. On the Acela train from Washington to DC, Susan and I experience a long-overdue cathartic moment.

Susan's embrace allows me to be truthful and open. We spend the next two hours talking about things we have never talked about before—on the frigging train! Deep conversation. I do my best to explain why I was afraid to let her know about the play. She is not angry. She does not, as I feared, yell, "How dare you?" Susan's inner strength and beauty are real, not the fictional fears of a fragile being I created in my head. She is and always has been steadfast and honest, the stoic and determined Susan I married.

Susan becomes a partner in the theatrical process. She laughs as we tell Ken and Ginny about the "Acela reveal." It becomes just one more crazy Sam story.

I now regret that Susan cannot stay for the reading. I have about a quarter of the script committed to memory. I also learn that one of the first theater professionals ever to hear the story—a New York producer of ballet—will be in attendance.

As soon as the reading ends, the professional's hand pops up. She has something to say. I hold my breath. "Sam, I want to compliment you on one thing right up front. One of the hardest things in playwriting or any new piece is the title, and I think you have hit it perfectly: "The Actual Dance." The comment builds my confidence.

The last reaction that night, though, is different and teaches me something fundamental about the story I tell. The group assembled in the large apartment has already dispersed into various rooms for snacks and informal chatting. I notice that Nadja, a colleague in New York who supports my work at Intersections, has not moved from her seat. Nadja is unique in her passions and life work, a recently ordained non-denominational minister, and a highly successful professional at a Wall Street firm. She is tearful. I sit down next to her.

"Are you alright?"

"Sam, I didn't know what this was about! I wish you had told me. I would not have come. I was diagnosed this morning with breast cancer."

I want to cry. I am surprised and shocked, and angry at myself. Why didn't I even think to let people know about the content of the show? The moment feels akin to what it would have been like if I had told Susan that I believed she would die during her treatment—something I took great care never to do. Now, what have I done?

Thankfully, Nadja has learned to love the show, while I learned an important and valuable lesson: the play and my performance will have an unknowable emotional impact on audiences. The truth is that until now, I have not confronted the depth of the emotional impact inherent in the story I am privileged to tell. Nadja's reaction was an early caution for me. Should there be a warning of some sort for audiences? As I discover more about producing theater, I learn that almost all theaters ask if the content should be limited to 'mature audiences' and we always say *yes*.

I have also learned that I cannot control how our audience experiences the show. A small number of those in attendance sometimes leave the theater in mid-performance. Most though, find a gift, sometimes a painful one, in my play.

CHAPTER 24

Us

The Actual Dance, the play, begins to transform audiences as it continues to change me. The words are written and spoken as if from me, to me. I am trying to solve a puzzle that sits unfinished on the table in the living room of my heart for nearly a decade.

Susan now attends many of the performances and joins me during the post-show dialogue with the audience. She expresses her experience of the same period, something I cannot do and which the play does not attempt. Her story is one of determination to survive. No, she did not know how I was feeling at the time. Indeed, neither did I. It took me a decade to begin to understand my own experience and to express it in the only form I could, a play. These shared experiences bring us closer together as we continue to develop a more profound love for each other. I feel compelled to acknowledge that I have been saying this repeatedly in this memoir. That's because I learn something every day about the idea of love.

As we begin to tour the play, I learn that I have missed something in Susan, a silent beat that I don't pick up because my band plays so loudly. I've created a company to produce The Actual Dance. I have an agent who is helping book the show, and I cannot perform enough. My ongoing discoveries in reliving these trying times are sometimes overwhelming, built on the audiences' reactions and stories. I begin to believe that my purpose in life is to bring The Actual Dance to all those who need to see it. Susan's story is different, and it takes a couple of whacks on the side of my head to understand.

As we approach our forty-ninth wedding anniversary, I propose to Susan that we rent the local community theater venue and invite the community and our friends and family to a performance, with a reception and party to follow. I love celebrating this way—telling the story about Susan's breast cancer and how it has led me to understand the true meaning of love. In response, she begins to cry. "Why are you crying?"

"I don't want to hurt your feelings. I just do not want to spend another anniversary reliving that story. I want us to celebrate, laugh, and have fun."

I feel so stupid. *What a fool. How blind can I be!* The light finally goes on in my brain.

"Oh, Susan, I am so sorry. Of course, let's celebrate in a way that brings both of us joy."

We spend a romantic weekend at a charming lodge, which sits on property once owned by George Washington, in Charleston, West Virginia.

The second reminder comes just a few months later. The Smith Center for Healing and the Arts, a nonprofit Washington DC cancer organization that hosted a performance a few months earlier, is now collaborating with the American University film and theater department to produce a video of stories about confronting cancer. Would Susan and I agree to sit for a video and tell our story?

"Yes!" I immediately respond. "I will confirm with Susan, and I just know she'll love it!"

I drive home from the Smith Center, pull into the garage, and burst into the kitchen, much the way I did some fifteen years earlier at the beginning of this story. Back then, she spoke first, telling me that everything in her annual check-up was fine, except the doctor had felt something funny in her right breast.

Today, I speak first. "Susan, guess what! The Smith Center wants us to do a video about our breast cancer experience and The Actual Dance. It won't take long."

She is at the kitchen sink washing something. In my memory, everything seems to slow down, a slow-motion unfolding of "The Susan." She turns her head toward me, then deliberately turns back to the sink, looking at what she is doing. I stop, frozen in my expectancy, waiting for the 'Yahoo! Let's do it." Nothing. Long pause. Finally, she turns around and, in a voice that is unmistakable in its perceived truth, exclaims, "Sam, I do not have cancer!"

I don't move. Again, I am alone in the center of a dance floor in a dark, empty-except-for-me ballroom, waiting for the orchestra that I know one day will form, as I think, *Oh, Susan, just, for now, my love. Just for now. Don't you know where I am?*

Snapping back to reality, I look at her and wonder why she doesn't ever listen, as I do. I listen—I listen with my heart where my love sits—for the ever-so-slight change in the balance of the universe that will indicate that a new and different orchestra has formed.

Yes, we sit for the interview. The students create a short video for a public program at American University that teaches students how to document community through story. We will be one of about six interviews.

Susan and I settle in for the shoot. We tell the story of her determination and my fears. The filming ends. Everyone in the room is off packing up while Susan and I remain in our chairs, waiting for someone to remove our microphones. A young woman, Becky, a college senior about to graduate and a member of the film crew, notices that the three of us are alone. She tentatively steps over to us and, in almost a whisper, asks, "What is your secret? I have never heard or felt such love and commitment between any two people."

A glance between Susan and me confirms that we both are perplexed by her unexpected question. The temptation, of course, is for me to reply: "The secret is, 'yes dear.' "

The young woman's voice sounds urgent. We sense we should not joke. She is serious and nervous. An answer pops to mind, something new and not well-thought-out.

"We promised each other," I say tentatively and eye Susan, who immediately knows where this is going. She nods her head and repeats. "We made a promise."

"We made a promise under the *chuppah* to love and honor the other forever. In sickness and in health. For richer or poorer. A sacred promise. A promise that we are not allowed to break. Even in the darkest times of a relationship, and there will be dark times, this promise to each other must be kept."

We learn something about ourselves from the spontaneity of that answer. We know that marriages do not always work out. We have seen throughout our lives people who find reasons to break that promise. We saw it in law school, as many of our married classmates suddenly discovered they wanted or were entitled to someone or something more. We saw it later in life, as even famous people left an ailing spouse for a newly discovered relationship.

The answer, or perhaps the question itself, is more challenging, hard to explain. Maybe the real "secret" we have revolves around a sense of an inevitability to our relationship, that Yiddish word "b'shert." *Meant to be.*

Yes, saying we are *b'shert* sounds corny and often leads to eye-rolling. The answer is not a map drawn by a marriage therapist. It is almost anti-intuitive. Success is what happens when we tough it out. Maybe too, it occurs when the fragility of life itself confronts us. A secret combination that we discovered through experience.

Our life together grows more beautiful and more vital every day. We continue to confront our existential challenges. We are more than ever as one together as we enter the last quarter of our lives—seventy-five years old as of this writing—living in a global pandemic. Our children are mid-career, indeed what used to be called midlife, each with responsible positions. They are principles in businesses that require them to face much more challenging moments than we do now. We have four grandchildren.

We talk about our time of life, two seventy-five-year-old people, and the future that confronts us. We are members of the oldest living generation of both families. We face a growing number of losses within our families. Susan's brother Buddy, my first cousin Sam Kobren, and my cousin Betty Anna have died within the last two years. Our generation is fading. We, Susan and Sam, have developed an inner spiritual strength to engage in moments of loss. Of anticipated loss. Of fear of the deaths of people we love most in the world.

We have already experienced moments of beauty and grace, of holding loved ones as they exit this world. We know that with each loss, we will start a new journey of transformation. We live in the world differently. Our purpose grows through these times as we realize that we must also live our lives in their honor. Their legacy becomes embedded in our actions and gifts.

Our journey, our actual dance, and the ritual of getting ready may have enabled us to prepare for these times. Susan's oldest brother died in 2019. In 2020, through the pandemic, the losses continued. A close cousin, a dear friend, and the most intimate friend of my adult life are all gone within one year. Susan and I stand with the ten people allowed to be at the burial ceremonies. We speak words of honor about our loved ones and try to comfort the rest of the family at their homes, watching over video.

Our journey in life, Susan and mine, is incalculably more meaningful, intimate, and connected. We have a relationship neither of us could have imagined. We have discovered the ability to be as one. Words I found when writing the play become animated in our lives every day: *I am the other half of that which makes us, Susan and me, complete.*

Three entities exist in our lives: Susan, Sam, and *us*. We are one sacred being. We are a sacred entity, entwined so intimately that we are the spiritual half of the whole. Nothing separates us.

Our discovery of *"us"* has gifts and challenges. It provokes and establishes genuine empathy for those in our circle of friends and family as they go through losing their loved ones. It also confirms my own experience, my continued periodic terror of losing the other half of my whole.

Yes, I believe that moment—when it comes—will be the ultimate consummation of our love in an ecstatic instant as the united souls are once again separated. In the pain of the end, we find the truth of the journey.

I wonder if we can ever be ready for the moment. As Susan and I discover even greater intimacy through these extraordinary moments of a pandemic, I wonder if I'm not just fooling myself. The hubris of thinking that I now know how to think about and experience the moment, should it ever arrive, is perhaps just ego.

I no longer pray that Susan not predecease me. I can't imagine either one of us having to bear that tearing asunder of *us*, of Susan and Sam.

I still imagine that moment of grace—the moment I now describe as a moment of beauty and dignity—that moment that defines what love means.

Susan and I embrace in a perfect waltz dance pose, together in a luminous ballroom, a place that only we experience. In a different dimension of space and time, we begin to glide gracefully throughout the room, passing by everyone we have ever met, have ever known, have ever loved in our lives, everyone from the generations before us, and yes, even generations yet to come. Somehow, we exchange a goodbye as Susan transforms into a

*wisp of white cloud and escapes my embrace into
eternity.*

So yes, every day, I listen. I listen with my heart where
my love sits for any indication that a new orchestra has
been called to play the song that only Susan and I can
hear.

Is that them playing?

Is that them playing?

Is that the orchestra playing our song?

GRATITUDE

(AKA: Acknowledgements)

*I*n reflecting on this last element of this work, I find using the word "Acknowledgement" inappropriate. The term is oddly neutral. We can acknowledge wrong conduct and sloth as well as love and generosity.

I prefer the word gratitude. My goal is to express my deep appreciation for the generosity of spirit and profound teaching, expertise, and loving support of the many people associated with The Actual Dance. The journey, which spans years, started with the discovery of the story hidden in my soul. Then came the writing and stewardship of the play and its performances. Now this book.

It is not possible to mention everyone. I urge you to visit the website for The Actual Dance to get a more detailed and full recognition of so many others, especially those associated with the elements of creating a theatrical production. www. theactualdance.com So, here is my attempt at the big thank you and, of course, we know where it starts.

Susan Simon, "the other half of my whole." I do not take Susan's participation in this journey for granted. Indeed, initially, I was afraid to tell her about the play I was writing, fearful that she would push back. Instead, in her classic loving way, she has embraced the journey. It isn't always easy, having to relive her illness. Yet, she lovingly supports me, attends most of the play's performances, and reads drafts of the book's manuscript. We now share a common vision of bringing this story to all who need to read it, so they too might imagine how to find "beauty and dignity" in life's worst moments. I am grateful beyond words for her love and gifts of generosity.

The Creative Team:

Gabrielle Maisels (gabriellemaisels.com). Of the many talented people who enabled me to discover and articulate The Actual Dance, Gabrielle stands first. Maybe she and I were supposed to find each other. Gabrielle started as my dramaturg, the person who guides the playwright in the creation of the story of the play. I still remember that evening in 2012, in New York, when she said, "Give me what you got." I read the draft, and she said, "You know, that was just fifteen minutes." Then she started asking questions. Gabrielle is a New York City-based solo show actress and an expert in "on-the-breath" acting techniques. She continues this journey with me, now directing the Zoom version of the play. She is also my acting coach. I know how rare it is to find long-term relationships that are both professional and personal. I am deeply grateful for Gabrielle's presence in my life, and her loving and professional talent has enlightened so much of this journey.

Carol Fox Prescott (carolfoxprescott.com). The person who connected Gabrielle and me with whom I continue a loving and learning relationship. Carol is the author of Breathing, Awareness, and Joy. She taught me to find the joy of my own experience and how to listen to my breath. Carol continues to be an essential presence in my life and artistic work.

Artistic New Directions (ANDTheater Company) (andtheatrecompany.org). I discovered the story that became this book through the gifts of a team of professionals who worked under the nonprofit Artistic New Directions Theater Company umbrella. I found AND, whose mission is supporting emerging actors, in the early 2000s and began attending their summer retreats in the Catskills to learn improv. Yes, Gabrielle and Carol were among those people I met through AND. I also want to mention many others, especially **Gary Austin, Jeffrey Sweet**, and **Kristine Niven**.

Jeffrey Sweet, himself a very successful playwright and author, introduced me to the technique of "improvising a story, writing it down, and performing it." I started doing just that, and what emerged was the story of The Actual Dance. But not right away. I kept trying to figure it out and worked with **Gary Austin**, the founder of the Groundlings in Los Angeles and perhaps one of the preeminent improvisers in America. Before he passed away, Gary was able to see the show—in tears. He told me he loved me and the show, giving me the gift of confidence to continue. **Kristine Niven**, who was the artistic co-director for Artistic New Directions throughout this period, and even now, is a fan of this work and has facilitated the emergence of the play in New York.

The Rev. Robert (Bob) Chase and the Collegiate Church of New York (intersections.org). My ability to engage in the New York sort of life, developing and discovering The Actual Dance, was based on the fortune of being invited to be Senior Fellow with Intersections International, a then brand-new social ministry of the Collegiate Churches of New York. They had hired as its director a friend of mine, The Rev. Robert Chase, who worked in the leadership of the United Church of Christ and was introduced to me by another mentor, the Rev. Dr. Everett Parker. At Intersections, I learned about the power of the arts to persuade people and unite a disparate world. Robert Chase's vision of working for justice along the thin edge of sharp differences, and using theater and music to do that, continue to be fundamental in my commitment to this journey. He and the Church have been very generous in supporting the developmental stages of The Actual Dance and then bringing a performance to each of their congregations. Mostly, though, I thank Bob Chase for introducing me to The Rev. Gregory Johnson.

The Rev. Gregory Johnson. I can still remember that first lunch with Greg, an adjunct minister at Marble Collegiate Church in New York. He was also the full-time director of a program at EmblemHealth, a major health insurance company in that city known as Care for the Family Caregiver. Greg immediately helped me understand something I didn't realize. I had been a "family caregiver" in my journey through Susan's cancer. His joy and generosity in all he does was an inspiration to me. He began to refer to The Actual Dance as "another face of family caregiving." He has perhaps attended more performances than anyone other than Susan and has generously secured financial support and bookings for performances in New York and beyond. His enthusiasm is infectious, and he brings unique insight not only in the theater but also in my understanding of what this love story means to so many others. Thinking about all the beautiful things he has done, one stands out—you know, the little things. We were about to start the New York run of the play at Theatre Row, an off-Broadway venue in Manhattan. He arrived early, came to my dressing room with a shoeshine kit, and reminded me how important it was for shoes to look sharp! I still look down before I go on stage anywhere.

So Many Others:

There have been so many other generous and kind people who helped me make this journey. I have traveled from an actual life event to a play, and now this book. I want to thank and acknowledge **Jessie Roberts** and her husband, **Jon Roberts**, my first director and sound designer. Their work resulted in my New York International Midtown Theater Festival performances with a nomination for best playwright and best sound. And in Northern Virginia, at the One-Act Festival, we won the award for the best original production. **Kate Holland**, my second director, took the theatricality of the play to a new level. She envisioned music and brought us Eli Katz Zoller, whose talent and musicality changed how deeply the play is received.

The generosity and support of so many people deserve mention. **Janie and Joe Roher**, for example, friends from days serving on the Board of Overseers (now called the Board of Advisors) of Hebrew Union College, have hosted Susan and me in their apartment many, many times. Living in McLean, Virginia, and being an actor in New York isn't easy! The executive director of Theater Resources Unlimited (TRU) in New York introduced me to **Joan Liman**, who allowed me to use an apartment for an entire month during our New York run!

The Book:

Linden Gross (lindengross.com). So how do you write a book of a story that I wrote as a play? You would think that a guy who had three books under his belt, including a book picked up by Book Of The Month Club as a premium gift when that was a thing, would know how to do this. Well, not so much. I pat myself on the back for finding Linden Gross, whose supportive and innovative style has carried me into transforming the play into an actual story in this book. Patience, support, and discipline adapted to my crazy style have gotten me to the finish line and across.

Lieve Maas (https://www.linkedin.com/in/lievemaas). A book designer with a great artistic eye, Lieve created a stunning cover that hopefully speaks to readers as much as it does to me. **Keri-Rae Barnum** (newshelves.com). Keri's deep knowledge of publishing helped get this book organized and out there!

About the Author

*S*am Simon describes *himself as being engaged in* his fourth age of life, as a playwright and performer. He likes to say that this era of his life found him, as did the story of *The Actual Dance* itself, after his wife was diagnosed with stage-three breast cancer.

Although Sam is a seasoned writer and author, he's an unlikely playwright and performer. He started as a lawyer committed to America's consumer movement. He was an original participant in Ralph Nader's first legal advocacy group, The Public Interest Research Group in 1970. He and his work have been featured in national media, including *The* New York Times, The Washington Post, Face the Nation, Good Morning America, Today, *The Phil Donahue Show, The Oprah Winfrey Show,* and other outlets. He is the author of two books and multiple articles.

In the late 1990s, Sam was introduced to and trained in theatrical improv at Artistic New Directions, now AND Theater Company in New York. He became a community member of Gary Austin's Workshop in New York and Washington, DC.

He wrote the play, *The Actual Dance,* which inspired this memoir, in 2012 and began performing in 2013. Since then, the play has been performed hundreds of times. The book and the play are autobiographical.

Learn more about Sam and connect with him at www.theactualdance.com.